HEAD AND
FACE PAIN
SYNDROMES

HEAD AND FACE PAIN SYNDROMES

RENE CAILLIET, M.D.

Professor Emeritus and Chairman
Department of Physical Medicine and Rehabilitation
University of Southern California School of Medicine
Los Angeles, California

Illustrations by R. Cailliet, M.D.

 F.A. DAVIS COMPANY • Philadelphia

Printed in the United States of America

Last digit indicates print number: 10 9 8 7 6 5 4 3 2 1

acquisitions editor: **Robert G. Martone**
production editor: **Gail Shapiro**
cover design by: **Donald B. Freggens, Jr.**

Library of Congress Cataloging-in-Publication Data

Cailliet, Rene.
    Head and face pain syndromes / Rene Cailliet:
illustrations by R. Cailliet.
       p.   cm.
    Includes bibliographical references and index.
    ISBN 0-8036-1625-2 (softbound: alk. paper): $22.00
(approx.)
    1. Headache. 2. Orofacial pain. 3. Migraine. I. Title.
    [DNLM: 1. Face. 2. Headache. 3. Pain.
WL 342 C134h]
RB128.C35 1992
616.8′491–dc20
DNLM/DLC
for Library of Congress   92-9879
                                               CIP

Preface

The complaint of head and face pain is heard daily by the general practitioner, and much confusion exists as to its true etiology, pathophysiology, mechanisms, and appropriate therapy.

In a 1985 national study conducted for Nuprin by Louis Harris & Associates Inc. of all the complaints of pain presented to the physician, listed under the heading of Hassles Scale, 82% of the high scorers suffered from headache as compared to 67% with low back pain, 63% with muscle pain, and 35% with dental pain.

Most of the medical literature written today is in the specialty of neurology, where major research currently occurs. These articles are read principally by neurologists and trickle down to the practitioner, as is true in most other specialties.

The American Association for the Study of Headache has emerged to address current research dealing with the daily care of the patient suffering from headache. Membership in this association has increased annually, indicating the burgeoning interest in this subject as well as indicating the magnitude of the problem.

The numerous theories of the etiology, mechanism, and treatment of headache remain controversial. Hippocrates wrote about migraine and its aura 2400 hundred years ago, and the controversy as to its being vascular or neurological remains unresolved. Treatment, therefore, has also remained ambiguous.

The somatic nervous system was originally considered the major pathway. More recently, the sympathetic nervous system has emerged as significantly pertinent, and as knowledge of the autonomic nervous system is further studied, its relationship to numerous head and face pain syndromes becomes more apparent and clarified. Neuropharmacological, endocrinological, and neurophysiological aspects appear more prevalent and better understood.

Migraine, migraine equivalents, and cluster headaches comprise the greatest interest and research for neurologists; but the chronic daily headache and neuralgias of the head and face present the greatest challenge to the average practitioner.

Fibromyalgia is a prominent concern of the pain patient seen daily by family practitioners, orthopedists, rheumatologists, physiatrists, and physical therapists, but its relationship to head and face pain has not been emphasized. As there is a strong relationship of fibromyalgia to head and face pain, it is fully addressed in this text.

The cervical spine and its pathology as a specific entity has been thoroughly studied by the medical profession, but the association of headache to the cervical spine remains controversial. This association is explored thoroughly as is full evaluation of recent research of this aspect.

The posttraumatic head pain syndromes become more prominent as the incidence of vehicular, sports, and military injuries increase. This presents a significant concern to the sophisticated patient so injured and frequently confronts the average physician. The legal aspects of this entity are also prominent in today's society and are fully discussed in this presentation.

The TMJ syndromes pervade the literature of the lay person and often cause excessive concern with overtreatment because of its lack of understanding. Although concept of myofascial pain is controversial, its presence is ubiquitous, and it is often inaccurately diagnosed and treated. Its significant relationship to TMJ pain syndromes is proposed and supported in this text.

The psychological aspects of head and face pain frequently confront the daily practitioner. The relationship of the psychological to the organic is fully recognized and thoroughly evaluated in this text.

The addition of this subject to the CAILLIET PAIN SERIES is an attempt to recognize the prevalence and significance of head and face pain as well as the previous consideration of other numerous musculoskeletal system disorders. It is the hope of the author to educate the practitioner in recognizing head and facial pain and postulating an appropriate understanding of the basics involved, postulating a more meaningful diagnostic work-up, and reaching a more rational managment program.

RENE CAILLIET, M.D.

Reference

Harris, L. and Associates: The Nuprin pain report. A national study conducted for Nuprin, Study #851017, New York, 1985.

Contents

Illustrations

CHAPTER 1

Anatomy, Physiology, and Pathophysiology of Head and Face Pain

In order to determine the source of pain emanating from the head and face we must ascertain the nerve pathways of the painful stimulus and the chemical and hormonal agents involved. In the past, head and face pain was thought to arise primarily from the somatic sensory system, but in more recent conceptualizations the sympathetic nervous system is becoming more prominent as a major pathway. The pathophysiology of migraine, for example, has been ascertained to be vascular, but there is now controversy as to whether migraine is a nerve-mediated syndrome rather than essentially vascular. As the vascular system is controlled by the sympathetic nervous system, there is obviously a direct relationship between the two. A semantic as well as conceptual difference exists.

Pain is known to be transmitted via somatic sensory nerves, a small portion of the motor nerve fibers, and a significant portion of the sympathetic nerves. All systems must be understood and their involvement discerned. There are many nerves in the head, neck, and face, but only the major nerves will be discussed here. For more precise and inclusive details readers may refer to pertinent texts.[1-3]

TRIGEMINAL NERVE

Pain in the intracranial and extracranial structures is subserved by cranial and upper cervical nerves. The trigeminal nerve is the Vth cranial nerve.

1

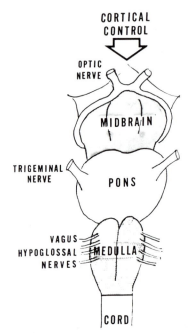

Figure 1–1. Midbrain, pons, medulla, and cord. The midbrain and the site of emergence of the trigeminal nerve from the pons is shown.

It is the principal innervator of the facial skin, cornea, oral and nasal mucosa, tongue, teeth, masticatory muscles, and meningeal lining.

The trigeminal nerve is the largest cranial nerve and is a mixed somatic sensory and motor nerve. It is a short nerve emanating from the ventrolateral surface of the pons (Fig. 1–1) and proceeding in an anterolateral direction to the apex of the petrous portion of the temporal bone (Fig. 1–2). At that point it expands to form the gasserian ganglion. The sensory roots are contained within this ganglion. The trigeminal nerve divides into three major branches, as shown in Fig. 1–2: the ophthalmic, the maxillary, and the mandibular.

The dermatomal areas of the face served by the trigeminal nerve are the face and anterior two-thirds of the head (Fig. 1–3). The motor roots, mentioned only for completeness, are also located within the pons beneath and below the sensory fibers and emerge via the foramen ovale at the point where it joins the sensory portion of the trigeminal mandibular division to innervate the muscles of mastication (Fig. 1–3).

Ophthalmic Division

The ophthalmic division is the uppermost and the smallest branch arising from the gasserian ganglion. It proceeds anteriorly through the wall of the cavernous sinus and through the superior orbital fissure to reach the

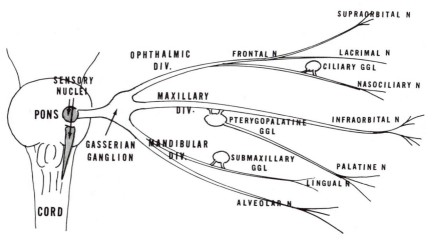

Figure 1–2. The trigeminal nerve.

The trigeminal nerve shown schematically has its sensory portion within the gasserian ganglion where the peripheral branches synapse to nerves entering the cord at the pons level to end in sensory nuclei. The trigeminal nerve branches into three major divisions: the ophthalmic, the maxillary, and the mandibular divisions. The sensory areas supplied by the trigeminal nerve are the face and the anterior two-thirds of the head. (See Fig. 1–3.)

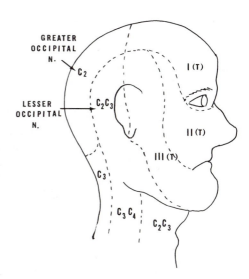

Figure 1–3. Sensory nerve supply to the face and head.

The branches of the trigeminal division, the occipital nerves through their branches, and the frontal nerves supply the skin of the head and the face. The trigeminal nerve divisions (TI, II, and III) are shown and the segments of the cervical plexus (C$_2$, C$_3$, and C$_4$) conveyed through the occipital branches are also depicted.

orbit. This division is exclusively sensory to the eye except vision and includes the conjunctiva, the lacrimal gland, the mucous membrane of the nose and paranasal sinuses, and the skin of the forehead, eyelids, and nose.

The ophthalmic division of the trigeminal nerve ultimately divides into three branches: the lacrimal, the frontal, and the nasociliary. The *lacrimal branch* supplies the lacrimal gland and the conjunctiva. It has postganglionic parasympathetic branchings, which are secretory motor fibers to the glands, and a significant sympathetic nerve supply. Any involvement of this division causes excessive lacrimation (tearing) and nasal congestion. The lacrimal branch anastomoses to the frontal nerve and the zygomatic branch of the maxillary division.

The *frontal branch* is the largest of the ophthalmic division. It enters the orbit via the superior orbital fissure. It supplies sensory input to the skin of the mesial lower portion of the forehead. Via its continuation as the supraorbital nerve, the frontal nerve supplies the upper lid and the mucous membrane of the frontal sinus. Involvement of this branch is probably the basis for many so-called sinus conditions. The frontal branch also supplies a portion of the scalp.

The *nasociliary branch* supplies the iris and the cornea with sympathetic supply to the dilator pupillary muscles. More precise details of these branches can be clarified in the medical literature.[1]

Maxillary Division

The maxillary division is the second division of the trigeminal nerve. It is entirely sensory, supplying the skin of the middle portion of the face: the lower eyelid, the side of the nose, the upper lip, and the mucous membranes of the nasopharynx, maxillary sinus, soft palate, tonsil, roof of the mouth, upper gums, and teeth (Fig. 1–2).

Near its origin it branches off to form the middle meningeal nerve, which supplies the ipsilateral middle meningeal artery and its branches to the dura mater; the dura mater is pain-sensitive within the cranium. The middle meningeal nerve divides into the infraorbital branch, which ultimately supplies the lower lid, the skin of the side of the forehead, the skin of the cheek, and the mucous membranes of the frontal, ethmoidal, and sphenoidal sinuses. One of its terminal branches, the greater palatine nerve, supplies the hard palate, the gums, the uvula, and a portion of the soft palate. The posterior superior alveolar branch supplies the gums, the mucous membrane of the cheek, and the molar teeth. Involvement of this division obviously is implicated in painful states of the midface, the lower orbit, and the nose and mouth structures.

Mandibular Division

This is the third and only mixed division; that is, it has both sensory and motor roots. Emerging from the pons region, the motor root passes beneath the gasserian ganglion and leaves the cranial cavity through the foramen ovale to rejoin the sensory components of the division.

The sensory fibers of the mandibular division innervate the skin of the temple area, auricula, the lower part of the face, and the external meatus of the ear, cheek, and lower lip. It also innervates the mucous membrane of the cheek, tongue, lower teeth, gums, temporomandibular joint, and a part of the dura mater and skull.

The motor branches of the trigeminal nerve supply the muscles of mastication: the masseter, temporalis, pterygoids, mylohyoid, and digastric muscles. All of these muscles are involved in opening, closing, and translatory motions of the mandible. This is obviously an important division in the identification and treatment of dental and temporomandibular arthralgia disease (TMJ) (see Chapter 6). The reader is encourged to refer to the literature for detailed branching and supply of this nerve division.[1,2]

The cutaneous afferent nociceptor fibers carried in the trigeminal nerve have been studied predominantly in the monkey, but a similar anatomical nerve supply has been ascertained in humans. Stimuli that damage or irritate the skin innervated by the trigeminal nerve traverse along small myelinated A-α and unmyelinated C-fiber nerves with free nerve endings. There are two types of A-α fibers: mechanosensitive receptors and A-α thermal nociceptor fibers.[4] The former require intense mechanical stimulus with resultant skin damage to respond. The latter respond to both mechanical and thermal stimuli, especially noxious heat. C-fiber nerves respond to chemical, thermal, and mechanical stimuli.

Pain occurs rapidly from noxious thermal stimulus, but a delayed pain response occurs when mechanical and chemical substances are released. Blood plasma releases pain-producing kinins, of which one is bradykinin. Bradykinin causes vasodilation and increased capillary permeability with resultant pain. Other substances are released from the extracellular fluid, including serotonin, which is algogenic. Mast cells are also released which in turn release histamine, also algogenic in high doses.

Trauma forms prostaglandins from breakdown (enzymic oxidation) of fatty acids: predominantly arachidonic acid. Many chemical and immunological stimuli activate phospholipids, which liberate arachidonic acid. Much occurs within the platelets that are liberated by trauma. The arachidonic acid ultimately breaks down into prostaglandins capable of causing pain.

Injury may also liberate substance P from cutaneous C nociceptors which also causes vasodilation and capillary permeability. The effusion following tissue injury also contains mast cells that liberate histamine: a potent vasodilator.

SYMPATHETIC NERVOUS SYSTEM

As pain is also mediated through the autonomic nervous system, a brief discussion of the relationship of functional anatomy to that of the somatic nervous system is pertinent.

The sympathetic division of the autonomic nervous system (Fig. 1–4) arises from preganglionic cell fibers located in the intermediolateral cell column of the 12 thoracic and upper 3 or 4 lumbar vertebrae of the spinal cord. After traversing the ventral roots they form the white communicating rami of the thoracic and lumbar nerves. From there they proceed to the ganglia of the sympathetic chain.

At the cord level the sympathetic sensory system, the somatic sensory system, and the somatic motor system merge (Fig. 1–5). The skin of the face and scalp receive sympathetic innervation from the superior cervical ganglia via plexuses extending along the branches of the external carotid artery (Fig. 1–6).

The neurogenic mechanisms that evoke vasodilation and constriction are poorly understood. Numerous neurotransmitters have been discovered, but none yet explain all aspects attributed to the vasomotor activity that underlies the various head and face pains of vascular etiology.

The classic transmitter acetylcholine and noradrenaline remain foremost as neurotransmitters of autonomic flow. The cerebral blood vessels are surrounded by nerve fibers that contain noradrenaline and neuropeptide Y, both of which cause vasoconstriction. The major purpose of this action allegedly is not so much to cause vasoconstriction but to attenuate excessive vasodilation created by the secretion of vasodilator substance P and neurokinin A, which are secreted by the trigeminal nerve.[5]

Acetylcholine is contained and liberated by numerous nerves surrounding major cerebral arteries.[6] It has been shown to cause relaxation of the blood vessels.[7] Whereas norepinephrine, acetylcholine, and vasoactive intestinal polypeptide (VIP) have been established as vasomotor neurotransmitters in the cephalic circulation, evidence is accumulating that there are numerous other neurotransmitters that are active.[8] Because head and face pain are closely allied to sympathetic and parasympathetic neurotransmission, much needed research remains to be done.

Syndromes Involving the Trigeminal Nerve

Lesions of the trigeminal nerve are usually termed *tic douloureux*. The patient experiences an excruciating pain in the distribution of one or more of the branches of the trigeminal nerve. This is discussed in detail in Chapter 4.

Syndromes involving the trigeminal nerve may be characterized by:

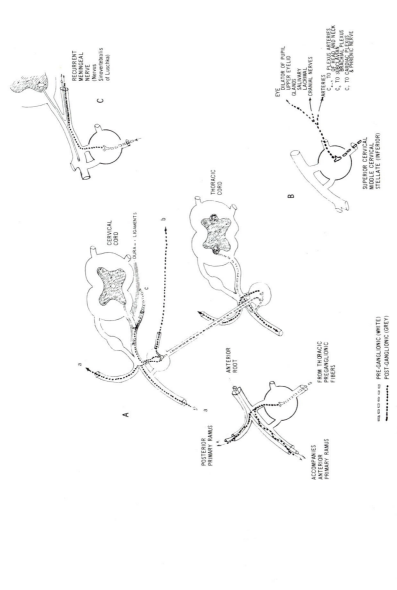

Figure 1–4. Sympathetic nervous system of the cervical region.

The autonomic fibers originate in the thoracic spine. The gray (unmyelinated) fibers leave the ganglia and course in three directions. (A) Along the posterior primary rami and anterior primary rami. (B) Through the superior cervical ganglia to the eye, cranial nerves, and arteries; and (C) Along the recurrent meningeal nerve to the dura and ligaments of the cervical spine.

7

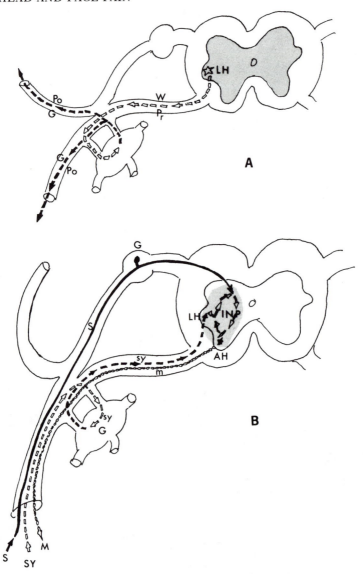

Figure 1–5. Sympathetic, somatic, sensory, and motor nerves at cord level.

(A) The direction of the sympathetic fibers in a segmental peripheral nerve is depicted. The autonomic fibers originate at the lateral horn cells (LH). (See Figure 1–4.) The preganglionic myelinated white (W) nerve (Pr), the postganglionic (Po) unmyelinated nerves leave as gray (G) fibers through the gray ramus of the ganglion (G) and proceed distally within the common peripheral nerve.

(B) The afferent pathways along the sympathetic nerve involve a cycle: The sensory nerve root (S) excites the internuncial pool (INP) which in turn excites the lateral horn cells (LH) of afferent sympathetic nerves (Sy) and afferent motor impulses (m). The motor impulses from anterior horn cells (AH) are both somatic and sympathetic.

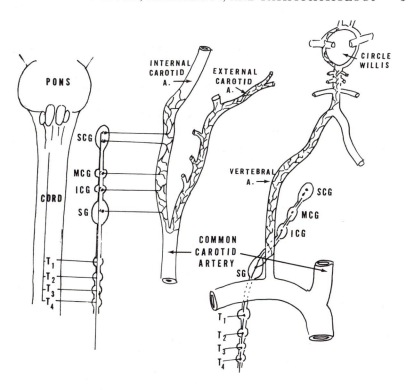

Figure 1–6. Sympathetic nerve supply to the head.

The preganglionic fibers originate from T_1, T_2, T_3, and T_4 segments of the cord and pass through white rami communicans to the paravertebral sympathetic chains, superior cervical ganglion (SCG), middle cervical ganglion (MCG), intermediate cervical ganglion (ICG), and stellate ganglion (SG) where they synapse into gray rami (postganglionic) to innervate the blood vessels of the neck and head.

The sympathetic fibers transmit autonomic motor fibers to the blood vessels and carry sensation from the peripheral areas.

1. Pain, which is marked to severe if the gasserian ganglion or its peripheral branches are involved.

2. Loss of sensation over the sensory distribution of the nerve and corneal anesthesia.

3. Dissociated anesthesia: Loss of pain sensation but not loss of touch, which implies involvement of the central spinal tract.

4. Paresthesia, indicating the possible involvement of the sympathetic nervous system.

5. Paralysis of the muscles of mastication, including deviation of the jaw toward the affected side.

6. Loss of jaw jerk and conjunctival and corneal reflexes.

7. Impaired hearing, implying paralysis of the tensor tympani.

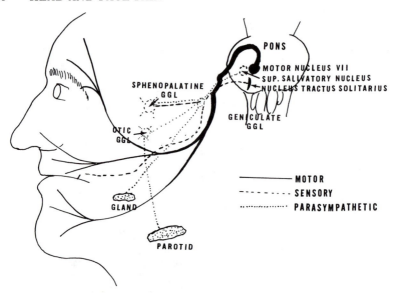

Figure 1–7. Facial nerve and its branches.

The central portion of the facial nerve (a mixed nerve in that it is sensory and principally motor) originates intracranially in the pons area. Here there exists the motor nucleus VII, the superior salivatory nucleus, and the nucleus tractus solitarius.

From the motor nucleus *(solid line)* emerge the motor nerves to the muscles of the face. From the superior salivatory nucleus emerge the parasympathetic nerves to various glands of the neck and face such as the parotid and the salivatory glands and to the nucleus tractus solitarius which enters the sensory *(dotted lines)* from the face.

The sensory patterns served by the facial nerve are periorbital, periocular, and nasal. The sensory fibers also carry taste fibers from the tongue.

The peripheral ganglia (optic and sphenopalatines) are sites of synapsis of sensory and parasympathetic nerves that are amenable to intervention in clinical impairments of these nerve fibers.

Clinically, the major pathological aspects of facial nerve involvement are motor (facial palsy), but the sensory components are of significant clinical importance.

8. Trismus or lockjaw, possibly brought on by rabies, tetanus, epilepsy, and hysteria.

9. Trophic and salivatory disturbances.

FACIAL NERVE

The facial nerve is a mixed nerve with a large motor component and a smaller sensory component (Fig. 1–7). The facial nerve originates from nuclei in the caudal portion of the pons. It initially loops around the nucleus of the abducens and ultimately terminates to supply the stapedius muscles of the middle ear, the muscles of facial expression, the platysma, and some muscles of the scalp.

The sensory portion of the facial nerve, with which we are more specifically interested, arises from unipolar cells that are innervated by fibers from the tractus solitarius within the pons. From the geniculate ganglion the nerve immediately divides into two branches. Their peripheral branches carry taste from the anterior two-thirds of the tongue via the lingual and chorda tympany nerves. The facial nerve also carries sensation from the parotid gland via the otic ganglion and the geniculotympanic nerves.

In its central connections the motor nucleus receives both contralateral and ipsilateral fibers from the corticobulbar tract, the extrapyramidal tracts, and the tectospinal tracts. The facial muscles innervated by the motor fiber of this VIIth nerve below the forehead receive contralateral cortical innervation and being bilaterally innervated, the frontalis muscle is not paretic or paralyzed by a lesion involving one motor cortex or its peripheral nerves.

Lesions of the facial nerve are primarily motor (75 percent of VIIth nerve involvements) causing a Bell's palsy (peripheral facial paralysis). The mouth droops and may be drawn toward the other side. Deep facial sensation is lost. Patient cannot whistle, wink, or close the ipsilateral eye. The forehead loses its wrinkles and the affected eye may tear excessively. On the sensory side the taste sensation of the anterior two-thirds of the tongue is lost, as is salivation on that side. Deep pressure in the neurological examination reveals a loss of proprioception of the facial muscles.

Lesions of the geniculate ganglion evoke an acute onset of pain behind and within the ear. Herpes is a frequent cause of this lesion. Lesions within the internal auditory canal may cause involvement of hearing (deafness) in that ear as the VIIIth nerve is in close proximity to the VIIth nerve at this site.

Lesions of the pons (for example, meningitis) may produce lesions of the VIIth nerve as well as the adjacent nerves: Vth, VIth, VIIIth, and XIth nerves.

In a nuclear type of facial palsy (see Fig. 1–7) there are signs of the peripheral palsy described above plus contralateral signs of hemiparesis.

There are numerous neurological syndromes associated with facial palsy of VIIth nerve etiology that are beyond the scope of this text and clinically are referable to a neurologist for consultation.[3]

CERVICAL NERVES

Each nerve root is composed of two roots: the anterior or ventral root and the posterior or dorsal root (Fig. 1–8). The former is principally motor and the latter is sensory. The roots are contained within a dural sheath (Figs.

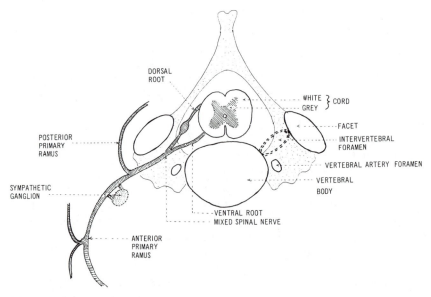

Figure 1–8. Cervical nerve root.

The dorsal root ganglion is within the intervertebral foramen and upon extra-cervical emergence it divides into posterior and anterior primary divisions. The sympathetic ganglia send autonomic fibers to both divisions. The vertebral arteries are shown lateral to the vertebral bodies.

1–9 and 1–10). The dorsal roots enter Lisauer's tract, which more recently has been designated as the layers of Rexed (Fig. 1–11). The dorsal root is three times thicker than the ventral root as it contains a greater number of axons.

In the cervical segments caudal to the upper cervical nerves[4] the nerve root emerges through the intervertebral foramina via "gutters" of the cervical vertebrae (Figs. 1–12 and 1–13).

In the upper cervical segment—the occiput-atlas and the axis—there are no foramina and no gutters. The nerve roots emerge through soft tissues (ligaments, muscles, etc.). The level of emergence from the cervical spine is numbered; C-1 emerges between the occiput and the atlas, and C-2 emerges below C-1 (Fig. 1–14). When the nerve roots emerge through the foramen and enter the gutter at the C-3 level, they occupy one-fifth to one-fourth of the foramen.

The dorsal ganglia of the sensory nerve root are located within the foramen at the lower segments, but in the upper cervical segment (C-1 and C-2) they are located above the vertebral arches near the vertebral arteries.

Of the cervical nerves the upper two roots pass laterally and slightly superiorly; C-1 passes between the occiput and the atlas (Fig. 1–15). C-2

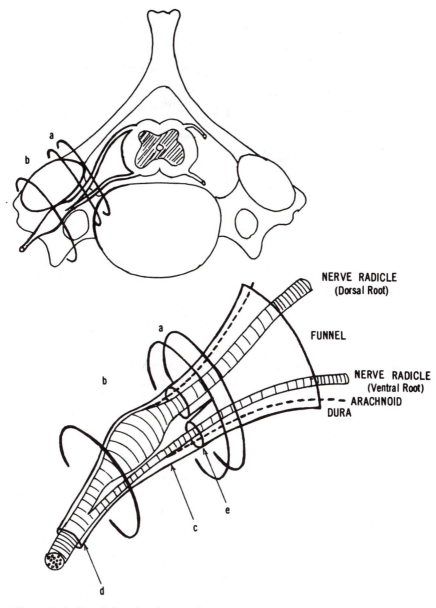

Figure 1–9. Dural sheaths of cervical nerves.

The dural-arachnoid sleeve of the cervical nerve roots in the intervertebral canal are depicted: (a) Intervertebral foramen is shown. (b) Gutter of the transverse process is shown. (c) At this point the arachnoid attaches to the dura and prevents spinal fluid from going farther. (d) The nerve from here on has only dural coating. (e) At the apex of the funnel (due to the inter-radicular septum) there are two ostia: One for the sensory and one for the motor roots. (From Cailliet, R: Neck and Arm Pain, ed 3. FA Davis, Philadelphia, 1991, p 34, with permission.)

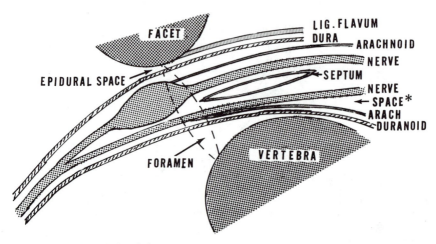

Figure 1–10. Dural sheath layers.

Schematic cross section of contents of intervertebral foramen depicts the layers of tissues lining the nerve roots as they emerge from the cord and enter the spinal canal. The ligamentum flavum lines the posterior inner wall of the spinal canal and ends at the facet area. The dura continues with the nerve root into the extraspinal region. The arachnoid space (*) contains spinal fluid. The space terminates at the orifice of the foramen.

passes between the atlas and the axis. Below this level, C-3 passes laterally anteriorly and causally within the gutter of the third cervical vertebra.

At the point where it emerges from the spinal cord each nerve receives several gray rami communicans nerves from the cervical sympathetic ganglia. The superior cervical ganglion contributes fibers to the upper four cervical spinal nerves.

As each nerve root emerges it divides into an anterior and a posterior primary division. The anterior primary divisions of the upper cervical nerves pass laterally behind the vertebral artery and unite to form the cervical plexus. The lower cervical roots unite to form the brachial plexus. Only the former are of significance in head and face pain.

CERVICAL PLEXUS

The anterior primary divisions of the uppermost cervical nerve roots unite to form the cervical plexus. Except for the first root (C-1) all roots divide into ascending and descending branches forming a series of loops. These loops are located lateral to the vertebrae and anterior to the levator scapulae and medial scalene muscles. They lie under the sternocleidomastoid muscles.

C-1, the suboccipital nerve, is the only branch of the posterior primary

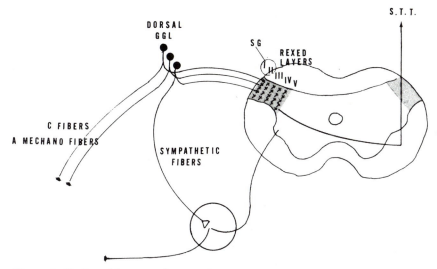

Figure 1–11. Rexed layers and sympathetic innervation.

The afferent C and A-δ fibers with their bodies in the dorsal ganglion (dorsal ggl) enter the gray matter of the dorsal horn of the spinal cord into the layers of Rexed I, II, III, IV, and V. Layers I and II are the substantia gelatinosum (SG). The sympathetic afferent fibers also enter the layers of Rexed carrying sensation. All ascend the cord to the thalamus via the spinal thalamic tracts (STT). (From Cailliet, R: Soft Tissue Pain and Disability, ed 2. FA Davis, Philadelphia, 1988, p 24, with permission.)

division. It has few, if any, sensory fibers and is primarily motor to the muscles of the suboccipital triangle.

The anterior primary divisions of the first four cervical nerves (C-1 to C-4) form the cervical plexus. The lower four (C-5 to C-8) form the brachial plexus (see Fig. 1–11). The small occipital nerve (C2-C3) supplies the sensation of the skin of the lateral occipital portion of the scalp, the upper aspect of the ear auricle, and the skin over the mastoid process. The great auricular branch (C2-C3) supplies the sensation of the skin behind the ear, the mastoid process, and the parotid gland. The cervical cutaneous nerve (also termed cutaneous colli) C2-C3 supplies the sensation over the anterior portion of the neck.

The communicating branches (not shown in the illustrations) communicate with the hypoglossial nerve from C1-C2 and carries motor function to the geniohyoid and sternothyroid muscles. They also supply sensation via sensory nerves to the dura of the posterior fossa of the skull via the recurrent meningeal branch of the hypoglossal nerve.

Lesions of the peripheral aspects of the upper cervical nerves are rare as they are well protected by the surrounding muscles. Tumors of the cord or meningitis are a common cause of upper cervical lesions. Upper cervical

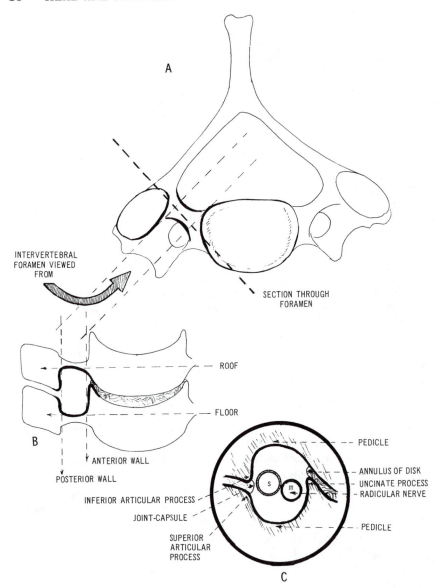

Figure 1–12. Anatomic borders of the intervertebral foramina.

(A) The boundaries of the foramen when viewed from the outside looking toward the spinal canal (large curved arrows) reveal the walls, roof, and floor as depicted in (B). The mixed nerve root (s = sensory, m = motor) is shown in (C). The proximity of the sensory fibers to the posterior articulations (facets) and the relationship of the motor to the Luschka joint and intervertebral disk is shown.

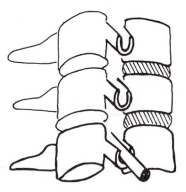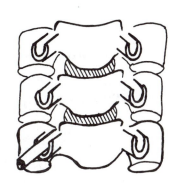

Figure 1–13. Direction of the foramenal gutters.

The gutter carrying the cervical nerve roots is directed in a downward and forward direction. (From Cailliet, R: Neck and Arm Pain, ed 3. FA Davis, Philadelphia, 1991, p 30, with permission.)

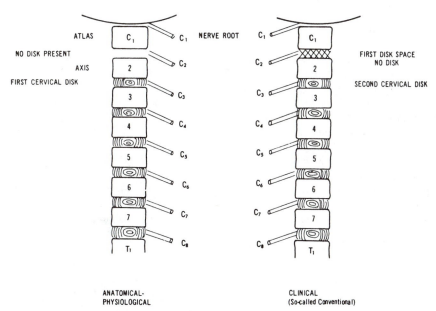

Figure 1–14. Nerve root location of emergence.

Nerve root level with regards to disk level. C_1 emerges above the C_1 vertebra between the occiput and the atlas (C_1). Anatomically there is no disk between the occiput atlas (C_1) and axis (C_2). (From Cailliet, R: Neck and Arm Pain, ed 2. FA Davis, Philadelphia, 1981, p 30, with permission.)

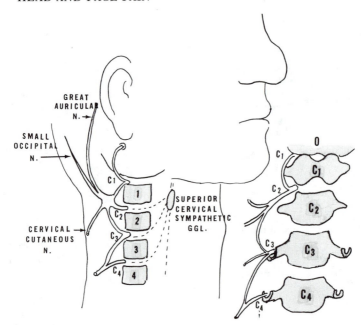

Figure 1–15. The cervical nerves.

The cervical nerves are derived from the cord segments that emerge between the occiput, the atlas (C_1), the axis (C_2) and the third cervical verebra (C_3). C_4 emerges between the C_3 and the C_4 vertebra. These nerve roots emerge from the spinal column in an anterior lateral direction. They are contained within the gutters of the cervical vertebra C_3 caudally. There are no gutters or intervertebral foramina in the uppermost cervical functinal units.

C_1 nerve (the suboccipital nerve) is the only branch of C_1 posterior primary division. It is mostly motor to upper cervical muscles.

C_2 nerve roots (along with a branch of C_3) form the great occipital nerve, which is sensory to the occipital portions of the back of the ear, mastoid area, and the parotid gland. The C_3 root sends branches to the C_2 root to form the small occipital nerve (C_2–C_3), which serves the skin of the lateral occipital portion of the scalp, the upper medial portion of the auricle, and the area over the mastoid process. It forms the third occipital branch and is sensory to a small portion of the scalp and neck. C_4 is sensory to the skin of the back and neck.

lesions may cause phrenic nerve paralysis with respiratory difficulty. Neuritis or neuralgia may occur from trauma, infections, metabolic disease, or psychogenic factors; they are felt in the occiput and upper cervical regions. These sensory nerves emerge behind the sternocleidomastoid muscle and branch up to the occiput (greater occipital nerve and lesser occipital nerve), forward and up to the ear (great auricular nerve), and downward and anteriorly to the anterior neck region (supraclavicular and transverse cutaneous nerves). These will be discussed in the specific pathological conditions.

AUTONOMIC NERVOUS SYSTEM

The autonomic nervous system supplies sensation as well as motor function to the vascular, lacrimal, and glandular function of the head and face. It is termed *autonomic* because most of its functions occur at the involuntary level.

The anatomy of the autonomic nervous system has been described earlier in this chapter; only pertinent factors will be repeated. The innervation of the blood vessels of the face and neck that probably are involved in migraine and cluster headaches are located in the columns of T-2 to T-4. These cell bodies in the intermediolateral columns receive descending fibers from diencephalic centers.

The axons of these fibers (myelinated preganglionic) emerge via the anterior roots of the upper four cervical nerves (C-1 to C-4); there they terminate in the cervical ganglia and they synapse with the cell bodies of the postganglionic neurones. The postganglionic fibers (mostly unmyelinated) outnumber the preganglionic fibers in a ratio of $32:1$. The postganglionic fibers then proceed to surround the common carotid artery, the external and internal carotid arteries, and the vertebral and basilar arteries (see Fig. 1–6).

The skin of the face and scalp receives fibers from the superior cervical ganglion via fibers from the plexus of the external carotid artery. The intrinsic muscles of the eye, salivary glands, and mucuous membranes of the nose and pharynx receive dual autonomic supply involving sympathetic, parasympathetic, and sensory somatic nerves.

The sympathetic nervous supply is affected by the emotions originally considered homeostasis or "flight or fight." In its action to the face and cranial viscera, vasoconstriction occurs peripherally, shifting the blood to the brain, skeletal muscles, and heart. Higher cortical control and the psychological aspects of head and face pain are discussed in Chapter 10.

Disorders of the autonomic system may lead to the following:

Horner's syndrome, which is a unilateral enophthalmos, ptosis, miosis, and a flushing of the face.

Acroparesthesia, which causes pain, hyperesthesia, hyperalgesia, and coldness of the hands.

Raynaud's disease, which affects the ears, toes, fingers, and tip of the nose. The parts are cold, pale, and cyanotic (bluish in color).

Causalgia, which is a painful condition of the hands and feet causing a burning sensation, hyperesthesia, swelling, redness, trophic nail changes, and ultimately the possibility of articular changes. The face and neck are not usually affected by causalgia, but facial changes are a possibility.

Migraine and migraine variants have a significant autonomic relationship that will be thoroughly discussed in subsequent chapters.

CEREBRAL AND EXTRACEREBRAL VASCULATURE

Many headaches have been attributed to vascular etiology: vasodilation or vasoconstriction. Pain has been elicited by stimulation of numerous vessels[11] both extracranial and intracranial (superficial temporal, supratrochlear, frontal, middle meningeal, superior sagittal sinus, and the sylvian vein). There are three major vascular systems supplying the head: (1) branches of the external carotid other than to the scalp, (2) branches to the scalp, and (3) the cerebral circulation.[12]

The branches of the external carotid other than to the scalp are predominantly to the face. The arterial supply to the scalp is derived from the superficial temporal artery. The scalp also receives branches from the supraorbital, supratrochlear, and ophthalmic arteries. The superficial temporal artery is clinically the most important.[13]

The meninges receive their blood supply from the external and internal carotids and the vertebral arteries. The brain receives its arterial supply from the vertebral arteries and the internal carotid arteries.

OROFACIAL PAIN

Acute pain in the face, head, and mouth frequently accompanies pathological conditions of the teeth and their associated structures. A thorough evaluation of a complex painful condition of the head and face should involve dental consideration. By properly coordinating the dental specialty proper diagnosis will evolve and the expectations from dental intervention will be more realistic. Analgesic injections may be diagnostic and ultimately therapeutic.

Dental involvement of temporomandibular arthralgia is considered paramount. This will receive consideration in Chapter 7. Mucosal pain disorders also must receive consideration. The oral cavity and anterior chamber of the nasal cavity are lined with stratified squamous epithelium, which has an abundant neurovascular supply and becomes a site of nociception. The mucosal disorders are numerous and may have a viral, bacterial, fungal, or mechanical etiology. These conditions are well discussed in the literature.[10]

CENTRAL MECHANISM OF PAIN TRANSMISSION

The preceding portions of this chapter have discussed the peripheral mechanism of pain transmission of the head and face. Free nerve endings are present in all the tissues of the face and head including the oral mucosa, temporomandibular joint tissues, peridontium, tooth pulp, periosteum, and muscles. The neurophysiological and psychological aspects of head and face pain are thoroughly considered in Chapter 11, but some neurological and anatomical aspects of pain will be considered here.

Sensations that will ultimately be considered pain are transmitted in small myelinated A-δ fibers and unmyelinated C fibers. The fibers are stimulated after injury by virtue of production of nociception mechanical, thermal, and chemical substances. The principal implicated chemical nociceptors are histamine, bradykinin, serotonin, potassium, and substance P. Tissue breakdown of arachidonic acid into phospholipid and then into prostaglandins is well documented in the rheumatology literature.

The peripheral nerves subserving the head and face enter the pons region via the Vth gasserian, semilunar ganglia, facial nerve, sympathetic nerves, etc. There are unmyelinated afferent fibers present within the Vth motor nerve but their function has not been elucidated. The Vth nerve component within the brain stem is extensive. It is considered the somatovisceral sensory nerve of the facial region. The afferents synapse with the two nuclei in the pontine gray matter: the spinal nucleus and the main sensory nucleus. The spinal nucleus corresponds to the dorsal horn of the spinal cord, and the main sensory nucleus corresponds to the dorsal column nuclei. In the spinal nucleus the afferents from mechanoreceptors, thermoreceptors, and nociceptors synapse with neurones sending axons to the reticular formation and/or the thalamus.

The reticular formation occupies a considerable portion of the brain stem. In addition to afferents from the Vth nerve it receives afferents from the spinoreticular tracts, propriospinal tracts, and most if not all the cranial nerves. Efferent impulses go to the thalamus, hypothalamus, limbic system, basal ganglia, and motor cortex, all of which receive afferents (Fig. 1–16).

SUMMARY OF NEUROLOGICAL ASPECT OF HEAD PAIN

The following summary factors will all be thoroughly discussed in the following chapters of the text.

Trigeminal neuralgia: Sudden, severe, brief, lancinating pain provoked by touch or movement of the facial areas innervated by the trigeminal nerve.

• *Ophthalmic division:* pain in forehead and supraorbital region and nose.
• *Maxillary division:* pain in the upper lip, cheek, side of nose, upper jaw, and teeth. Site of provocation is frequently the upper lip and occasionally the upper gums.

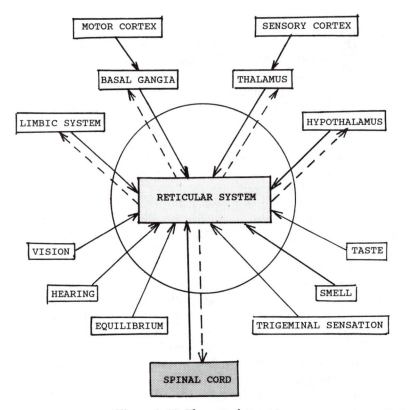

Figure 1–16. The reticular system.

• *Mandibular division:* pain in mandibular region, lower lip, chin, jaw, gums, and ear. Site of provocation is the lower lip.

• *Genicular neuralgia:* tic douloureux pain deep in the ipsilateral ear and postauricular area. Area of provocation is the inner ear: occasionally incited by swallowing.

• *Glossopharyngeal neuralgia:* severe lancinating pain in the tonsillar or pharynx area and back of tongue. Area of provocation is the throat: hence incited by swallowing and talking.

Occipital neuralgia: continuous aching, throbbing pain in the suboccipital area, the posterior and lateral scalp. Occasionally there is pain in the retro-orbital region. No specific area of provocation other than from deep pressure in the suboccipital area near the mastoid process.

Migraine headache: throbbing, pulsating, pressing pain. Usually the headache is unilateral. Often preceded by prodromal symptoms (aura).

Migraine variant: similar to migraine with predominance of neurological symptoms related to a specific cranial artery. No regional area of provocation.

Cluster headache: sudden unexpected unilateral aching or burning pain in ocular, frontal, and temporal area. No area of provocation.

Acute headache: severe continuous generalized headache with associated other symptoms: Provoked or initiated by meningitis, subarachnoid hemorrhage, cerebral vascular accident, or spinal puncture.

Musculoskeletal headache: characterized by temporomandibular arthralgia—dull aching pain in the muscles of mastication (chewing) provoked by movement of the jaw.

- *Myofascial pain syndrome:* dull aching deep muscular pain located within a specific muscle group. Provoked by pressure on a trigger point within that muscle.

Ocular or periorbital pain:

- *Ocular pain:* deep dull aching pain often with "foreign body" sensation.
- *Orbital pain:* deep dull aching pain in orbit often with lid edema.

Ear, nose, throat pain: Pain located in the specific organ (ear, nose, throat, paranasal, or frontal sinus). Local pain and tenderness of the region with associated symptoms of disease. Often evidence of inflammation or infection.

Pyschogenic pain: pain described in bizarre symptoms, vague etiology, poor neurological demarcation, and associated with other psychological factors.

REFERENCES

1. Bonica, JJ: The Management of Pain, Vol I, ed 2. Lea & Febiger, Philadelphia, 1990, pp 651–793.
2. Clemente, CD (ed): Gray's Anatomy, Am ed 30. Lea & Febiger, Philadelphia, 1985, pp 1158–1189.
3. Chusid, JG: Correlative Neuroanatomy and Functional Neurology, ed 14. Lange Medical Publishers, Los Altos, 1970, pp 98–101.
4. Dubner, R, Price, DD, Beitel, RE, and Hu, JW: Peripheral neural correlates of behavior in monkey and human related to sensory-discriminative aspects of pain. In Anderson, DJ and Mattews, B (eds): Pain in the Trigeminal Region. Elsevier, Amsterdam, 1973, pp 57–66.
5. Lundberg, JM, Hokfelt, T, Anggard, A, Terenius, L, Elde, R, Markey, K, Goldstein, M, and Kimmel, J: Organizational principles in the peripheral sympathetic nervous system. Subdivision by coexisting peptides (somatostatin-, avian pancreatic polypeptide-, and vasoactive intestinal polypeptides-like immunoreactive materials). Proc Natl Acad Sci USA 79:1303–1307, 1982.
6. Edvinsson, L, Owman, C, Rosengren, E, and West, KA: Cholinergic mechanisms in pial

blood vessels. Histochemistry, electron microscopy and pharmacology. Z Zellforsch 134:311–325, 1972.

7. Edvinsson, L, Falck, B, and Owman, C: Possibilities for a cholinergic action on smooth musculature and on sympathetic axons in brain vessels mediated by muscarine and nicotinic receptors. J Pharmacol Exp Ther 200:117–126, 1977.

8. Brayden, JE, and Bevan, JA: The autonomic innervation of the cephalic circulation. In Olesen, J and Edvinsson, L (eds): Basic Mechanisms of Headache, Elsevier, Amsterdam, 1988, pp 145–155.

9. Cailliet, R: Neck and Arm Pain, ed 3. FA Davis, Philadelphia, 1991, pp 30–31.

10. Eversole, LR: Mucosal pain disorders of the head and neck. In Jacobson, AL and Donton, WC (eds): Headache and Facial Pain. Raven Press, New York, 1990, pp 53–80.

11. Ray, BS and Wolff, HG: Experimental studies in headache. Arch Surg 41:812, 1940.

12. Dahl, E and Edvinsson, L: Anatomical organization of cerebral and extracerebral vasculature. In Olesen, J and Edvinsson, L (eds): Basic Mechanisms of Headache, Vol 2. Elsevier, Amsterdam, 1988, pp 24–47.

13. Gray, H: Anatomy of the Human Body. Lea & Febiger, Philadelphia, 1973.

CHAPTER 2

Migraine and Migraine Variants

Headache, probably the most common medical complaint of civilized humanity, is, surprisingly, rarely caused by organic disease. The complaint of headache is no longer simply considered a symptom but actually now can be categorized into specific disease entities. Among the leading etiologies of headache symptoms the vascular headache remains foremost, with migraine and its variants being preponderant. Other forms of headache also have gained acceptance as a specific disease entity, but migraine remains unquestionably unique.

Some 2400 years ago Hippocrates wrote about migraine and its aura. A century ago, William Osler postulated the etiology of migraine to tension in the muscles of the head and neck.[1] Neurologists have researched migraine headache intensely, and numerous theories have evolved. In 1963 the Ad Hoc Committee on the Classification of Headaches offered a standardized classification.[2] However, many clinicians feel this classification is useful primarily to researchers and academic proponents who want to establish the rationale for therapeutic drugs which have little value in daily clinical practice.

Vascular headaches termed migraine have been classified as classic and common migraine, hemiplegic migraine, ophthalmoplegic migraine, cluster headaches, and toxic headaches among other terms. All are classified by symptomatology as there are no significant diagnostic procedures that clarify the etiology or the type. What symptoms, if any, precede or accompany the headache determines whether the migraine is classic or common. All or most of the symptoms are attributed to a neurovascular etiology.

In essence, the differentiation between classic or common migraine depends on whether there is a prodromal aura phase in the headache. The patient's associated systemic complaints may further confuse or complicate a clear diagnostic differentiation. The neurological system implicated in the subjective complaint of the aura influences the classified diagnosis as is evident in such labels as ophthalmic, hemiplegic, toxic, etc.

The pain-sensitive structures within the cranium have been evaluated as to their relationship to the symptom of headache.[3] With clarification as to structure there has also arisen a question of which mechanism affects that particularly sensitive structure causing symptoms.

When ergotamine emerged as a significant medication for migraine the theories were reexamined. Since 1930 several concepts have unfolded.

1. Aura is the result of vasoconstriction of the cranial blood vessels.

2. The headache of migraine results from vasodilatation of the cranial blood vessels.

3. Ergotamine aborts migrainous headaches by virtue of its vasoactive properties. (This concept is more recently being challenged.)

4. There is a central basis for the autonomic activity resulting in peripheral vasomotor activity.

Harold Wolff,[4] a prominent researcher in migraine mechanisms, postulated and experimentally sustained the vascular concept of migraine. He claimed that migraine auras created by vasoconstriction could be ameliorated and even banished by amyl nitrate, a strong vasodilator. He also maintained that the benefit of ergotamine resulted from the vessel constriction, a condition that he was able to reproduce in his laboratory. He demonstrated the production of kinins, which chemically lowered the pain threshold; edema of the extravascular arteries by biopsy; and vascular instability between attacks.

Doubts emerged in the 1970s about the exclusive or predominantly vascular genesis of migraine. Laboratory studies of cerebral vascular flow did not correlate with symptomatology. Lauritzen and Olesen[5] demonstrated that during a migraine attack a band of vascular flow abnormality originated in the occipital region of the brain and spread forward at a rate of approximately 2 to 3 mm/min; this did not appear to be consistent with normal vascular action. These findings were confirmed by Lashley[6] and Leao,[7] who asserted that migraine was primarily neurogenic and the vascular component was a secondary related action.

It appears from the research that the verdict as to etiology—vascular or neurogenic—is not completely accepted. Both probably play a part in causing symptomatology, and both must be therapeutically approached. Table 2–1 shows the classification of migraine by the International Headache Society.

Table 2–1. INTERNATIONAL HEADACHE SOCIETY CLASSIFICATION OF MIGRAINE (1988)

1. Migraine
   - 1.1 Migraine without aura
   - 1.2 Migraine with aura
     - 1.2.1 Migraine with typical aura
     - 1.2.2 Migraine with prolonged aura (>1 hour <1 week)
     - 1.2.3 Familial hemiplegic migraine
     - 1.2.4 Basilar migraine
     - 1.2.5 Migraine aura without headache
     - 1.2.6 Migraine with acute onset aura
   - 1.3 Ophthalmoplegic migraine
   - 1.4 Retinal migraine
   - 1.5 Childhood periodic syndromes that may be precursors to or associated with migraine
     - 1.5.1 Benign paroxysmal vertigo of childhood
     - 1.5.2 Alternating hemiplegia of childhood
   - 1.6 Complications of migraine
     - 1.6.1 Status migrainosus (>72 hours)
     - 1.6.2 Migrainous infarction (symptoms/signs of aura >1 week)
   - 1.7 Migrainous disorder not fulfilling above criteria

MIGRAINE: CLINICAL FEATURES AND DIAGNOSIS

The symptom of headache is so prevalent that many physicians are disdainful of headache patients. The acceptance of migraine as being largely "emotional" in etiology evokes a feeling of despair and frustration in the treating physician. Headache must be placed within the global context of the patient's lifestyle—psychosocial, familial, dietary—and medical consideration must be given to other somatic complaints, reaction to medications, and so forth. All must be evaluated and placed into context in formulating a treatment plan for the headache patient. Merely to treat a migraine patient with a specific medication for the isolated attack will often fail in the long run.

The precise diagnosis of migraine must be confirmed by a meticulous history because the ensuing examination and laboratory confirmation is usually nonconfirmatory. The main purpose of a complete neurological examination and laboratory radiologic studies is to reveal other organic pathology that resembles a migrainous headache. The diagnosis of migraine must never be made unless:

1. There have been five or six similar attacks
2. An attack lasts at least 4 hours

3. The headache is unilateral (hemicranial)
4. There are elicitable prodromal symptoms (not necessarily aura)
5. There is no organic pathology

History

The history should include:

1. Family history
2. Age of onset of headaches
3. Location and quality of the headache
4. Duration and frequency of the headache
5. Medications and foods associated with onset
6. Associated symptoms, including prodrome and aura

Family History. Seventy-five percent of migraine patients have a first-degree relative who also has migraine.

Age of Onset. Classic migraine headache usually has its onset in adolescence or young adult life. Occasionally, migraines may begin in childhood or in later adult life, but these require careful evaluation to eliminate the possibility of other organic types of headache. Migraine occurs four times more frequently in females than in males.

Location of Headache. Characteristically a migraine headache is unilateral and has a throbbing quality. It can be best characterized by the patient as moderate to severe.

Duration of Headache. The migraine headache usually lasts several hours to a full day. Some have been reported as lasting 2 to 3 days. Rarely, a classic migraine headache may last over 72 hours, in which case it is termed *status migrainosus.*

Migraine attacks tend to recur two to three times a month and typically occur upon arising; they rarely awaken the patient.

Provocative Factors and Substances. Migraine can be elicited, provoked, or aggravated by changes in the patient's environment such as menstruation, sexual activity, minor head trauma, emotional stress, and even significant weather changes. These factors are elicited after an attack or as part of the patient's history.

Medications and certain food substances that influence the migraine are also diagnostic. Vasodilator medications such as nitroglycerin, reserpine, and amyl nitrate may incite an attack. Alcoholic beverages are also incriminated, as are processed foods containing nitrates, monosodium glutamate, hard cheeses, nuts, herring, chocolate, and caffeine. Occasionally attacks may be precipitated by citrus fruits. These drugs and foods alone are not diagnostic, but when added to the first criteria they are additional to diagnosis and also implicate substances to be avoided in preventative prescription. Many over-

**Table 2–2. INTERNATIONAL HEADACHE SOCIETY
CRITERIA FOR MIGRAINE**

A. At least two attacks fulfilling B
B. At least three of the following characteristics:
   1. One or more fully reversible aura symptoms, indicating cerebral cortical and/
      or brain stem dysfunction
   2. At least one aura symptom develops gradually over more than 4 minutes or
      two or more symptoms occur in succession
   3. Aura symptom lasts less than 60 minutes (if more than one aura symptom is
      present, accepted duration is proportionally increased)
   4. Headache follows aura with a free interval of less than 60 minutes. (It may
      also begin before or simultaneously with the aura.)
C. History and examination do not suggest an organic or metabolic disorder, or the
   latter is ruled out by appropriate investigations, or the migraine attacks do not
   occur for the first time in close temporal relation to an organic or metabolic
   disorder.

the-counter drugs that may be used with impunity often contain caffeine or
a vasodilator. These include sinus medication, cold remedies, cough medications, and so forth. Barbiturates, contraceptive drugs, and ergotamine have
also been implicated.

Adverse effects of drugs and foods are not criteria for diagnosis but are
supportive in affirming the diagnosis.

In a careful history of confirmed migraine patient all aspects of daily
living—stress, foods, drugs, etc.—must be explored and evaluated in a effort
to prevent attacks.

Associated Symptoms. Symptoms associated with migraine such as nausea, photophobia, phonophobia, abdominal cramps, pallor of face, and tenderness of templar blood vessels are frequent and are actually considered
essential by many clinicians to accurately diagnose the headaches as migraine
(see Tables 2–2 and 2–3).

**Table 2–3. CRITERIA FOR COMMON
MIGRAINE (ALBERT EINSTEIN COLLEGE OF
MEDICINE, NEW YORK)**

Recurrent idiopathic headache associated with at least
two of the following:
1. Nausea with or without vomiting
2. Unilateral pain
3. Throbbing quality
4. Photophobia or phonophobia
5. Increased by menses and a positive family history*

*Can be removed without altering the specificity
of the criteria.

The mechanism underlying migraine attacks remains unclear. There is some debate as to whether these prodromal symptoms merely precede the migraine or are in fact the initial phase of the attack.[8] The symptoms may continue, increase, or become modified during the attack and often persist after the head pain has disappeared.

These prodromal symptoms also vary as to which system is involved. They may involve the autonomic system with vasomotor sequelae, the neurological system, or the muscular system with spasm and muscle pain. The mental signs vary from excitatory to withdrawn, the muscular signs range from stiffness to weakness, and the gastrointestinal symptoms can vary from craving to anorexia. It is impossible to determine which symptoms are specifically linked to the attacks without a careful inventory by history. Their relationship follows in retrospect.

All symptoms vary from the normal through the prodrome, the active headache stage, the recovery, and often into the postmigraine normal. The neurological aspect of these symptoms have thus been used to justify the neurological etiology of migraine.[9]

Classic migraine is diagnosed when the prodrome is followed by an aura. Auras vary greatly and include visual, sensory, motor, or speech symptoms.[10] A typical visual aura follows the prodrome and precedes the headache by 20 to 30 minutes. The common auras are scotoma—a blind spot in vision— or an arc of scintillating flashing lights. The scotoma may begin as a circle of flashing light that increases in size gradually. Hideous patient drawings of these scotomas permeate the literature and are often used by pharmaceutical companies in their literature of recommended drugs. The presence of prodrome followed by aura without subsequent headache has been considered sufficient to diagnose migraine.

Besides the visual aura in classic migraine there are other auras that merit mention. Sensory auras are second in frequency to visual auras.

Sensory auras are usually a paresthesia, especially a sensation of numbness. They are usually a one-sided occurrence and tend to spread. In the upper extremity paresthesia of the thumb may spread to the whole hand and progress to the perioral area. Paresthesia may effect only the upper or the lower extremity, and the side may change in other attacks. Paresthesia may be the first sensation of the aura and be replaced by numbness of the involved area.

The peripheral aura may be the same side of the headache but variation occurs.[10a] The duration is also variable lasting from less than 1 hour to more than 7 days.[10b]

Motor aura may be weakness which develops focally and spreads to involve one or more muscle groups. The weakness may vary from a feeling of heaviness to a massive hemiparesis. The weakness may be in one extremity, in more than one extremity, or be bilateral. Motor weakness may accompany sensory aura or be related. There are various combinations reported.

Only visual aura may occur in isolation, but sensory, motor, or speech aura are usually associated with visual aura.[10d]

Physical Examination

A complete physical examination must be undertaken and appropriate laboratory tests undertaken. These tests, however, must be consistent and appropriate. If a thorough neurological examination reveals the possibility of an organic component, a lumbar puncture, a CT scan, or an MRI is certainly justified. However, only when there is a basis for these studies should the financial and emotional expense be imposed upon the patient.

Complete blood studies are warranted in a thorough medical evaluation. X-rays of the head, cervical spine, and temporomandibular joints are justified only when their interpretation will confirm and qualify the findings from the history and the neurological examination.

TREATMENT

Once the clinical diagnosis is confirmed by history and all other neurological organic aspects have been ruled out, the treatment is reasonably standardized. Unfortunately, in the opinion of many clinicians, it is only useful to treat the acute episode, as preventative treatment has not proven fruitful, and in some cases has even been detrimental. It behooves the clinician to review this concept.

Treatment begins with the history and physical examination, which must be perceived by the patient as personal, thorough, and appropriate. The psychological aspect of the history must be obtained early so that it is not viewed as an afterthought by the physician if all tests and treatments prove not to be beneficial. The relationship of emotional factors to head pain that has no apparent organic component must be explained early in terminology understood by the patient. If an explanation is not carefully worded, it can seem like an accusation, no matter how well-meaning the physician. A sympathetic explanation can mark the beginning of a meaningful relationship between physician and patient. All treatment aspects must be tailored to the individual personality of the patient, who frequently approaches the physician with preconceived ideas of causation, treatment, significance, and prognosis of the disease. Many patients have often utilized self-procured medications that may have been of no value or actually detrimental and addictive.

Compliance with treatment and medications for other conditions should also be evaluated to determine the expected compliance to the projected treatment initiated for this condition. Compliance as related to effective treatment and prevention of relapse or even failure of an adequate treatment program is undergoing intensive study.[11] Compliance and noncompliance will receive thorough evaluation in Chapter 11.

Nonpharmacological Treatment of Migraine

There are many somatopsychic as well as pertinent diagnostic subjective components in the complaints of the migraine headache patient. All should be considered.

The emotional components of migraine headache are well documented and should be addressed. If the patient history indicates that a given emotional situation may provoke a migraine headache, stress management, biofeedback, counseling, and even psychotherapeutic assessment may be advisable and beneficial. An explanation of the association between stress and migraine will often encourage compliance. Statements that the migraine is "merely" emotional will generally be regarded by the patient as an unhelpful rebuke. Sophistication on the part of the patient, no matter how educated, cannot be assumed. Posttraumatic stresses and tensions have been invoked as provocative and should receive attention.

Food sensitivities as migraine provokers have been postulated but not specifically confirmed. When these provokers are enunciated by the patients, they should be discussed and their elimination advised. A dietician may be of value in these conditions. It is important that patients not miss meals; the combination of stress, fatigue, and skipped meals may trigger a migraine attack.

Time factors have also been implicated in migraine attacks. Sometimes sleeping late on weekends seems to be the cause, particularly when regular awakening hours during the week are not provocative; hence a change of sleeping habits is of value. It is of interest that migraine appears to be less frequent on vacations than during regular daily activities, indicating a relationship of fatigue, stress, and tension. Vocational change may be indicated if migraine becomes intractable.

Pharmacological Treatment of Migraine

In the accurately diagnosed migraine headache, the earlier treatment is instituted, the better are the chances of aborting or minimizing the attack. The immediate ingestion of an analgesic such as aspirin, dextropropoxyphene, acetaminophen, or a codeine derivative may be all that is necessary. In addition, reclining in a dark room with an ice compress to the temple area should be instituted. In one study vigorous digital massage and compression of the superficial temporal arteries during the visual aura of an attack was found to be 80 percent successful.[12]

When debilitating migraine headaches, with or without aura, recur frequently, appropriate medications should be prescribed. Acceptance and efficacy of these medications must be ascertained as they tend to become the patient's medication of choice.

Certain drugs are more or less effective depending how they are administered. Patients who are especially prone to nausea and vomiting with a migraine attack may experience increased nausea with certain medications. The delay in the absorption of certain drugs taken by mouth also diminishes or even negates their being the drug of choice.

Ergotamine tartrate has proven over the years to be particularly effective when taken within the first hour or two of a proven attack. The route of administration here plays a significant role: ergotamine tartrate has proven 90 percent effective when given parenterally, 80 percent effective when given rectally in a suppository, and only 50 percent when given orally.[13] Ergotamine tartrate in high doses delays gastric emptying by its smooth muscle action and causes gastric irritation with epithelial damage.

Ergotamine is pharmacologically a smooth muscle stimulator, causing vasoconstriction. In the past the efficacy of this medication seemed to confirm the vascular etiology of migraine, but that is now being questioned. More recent studies have postulated a central nervous system effect and a peripheral adrenogenic mechanism.[14]

Ergotamine alkaloids comprise ergotamine tartrate and dihydroergotamine (DHE-45) and are available in various forms for different application: intravenously, intramuscularly, subcutaneously, orally, rectally, by inhalation, and as sublingual tablets. These alkaloids are currently available on the market in the following preparations (others may be added to the pharmacopia):

Cafergot tabs	1 mgm
Cafergot tabs PB	1 mgm
Cafergot suppositories	2 mgm
Cafergot suppositories PB	2 mgm
Wigraine tabs and suppositories	2 mgm
Ergomar sublingual tabs	2 mgm
Ergostat sublingual tabs	2 mgm

Some of these tablets contain caffeine, phenobarbital, and/or belladonna. These additive medications may be contraindicated for particular patients.

Ergotamine and related alkaloids are contraindicated in patients with significant hypertension, peripheral vascular disease, thrombophlebitis, ischemic heart disease, collagen vascular disease, or cardiac valvular disease. They must be carefully monitored in patients over 60 years of age and in patients with bradycardia, renal abnormalities, or peptic ulcer history. Caution should be exercised if the patient experiences nausea, vomiting, diarrhea, abdominal cramping, vertigo, or paresthesiae of the hands or feet (vasoconstriction) if brief (lasting an hour or less). These symptoms should be explained to the patient for reassurance and for reporting purposes.

Use of an ergotamine alkaloid in combination with other drugs must be monitored. Combination with a beta blocker may initiate excessive bradycardia; this may be alarming and potentially detrimental.

Susceptibility to ergotamine tartrate is infrequent but significant if present. Dependency has been reported in patients who utilized ergotamine as frequently as three times weekly. Patients have reported a "rebound" (headache) if the medication is discontinued or decreased or even after a third dose is taken. This dependency has been reported in patients taking ergotamine tartrate more than 2 days a week.[15]

Midrin (isometheptene mucate) is a specific migraine medication which does not contain ergotamine but which is effective in treating the acute attack. This medication is a sympathomimetic agent; it contains isometheptene (65 mgm), acetaminophen (325 mgm), and a tranquilizer (dichloralphenazine). It is indicated in milder attacks and causes less gastrointestinal irritation than ergotamine. In patients with nausea and vomiting it is effective.

Midrin is best prescribed as two tablets immediately upon an acute attack followed by one or two capsules 1 hour later. A maximum of five capsules per attack is recommended no more than 2 to 3 times per week, as it may also initiate a rebound effect.

Nonsteroidal anti-inflammatory drugs (NSAID) have a beneficial effect in an acute attack either alone or in combination with Midrin. NSAIDs are too numerous to mention in this text, but they and their side effects and contraindications are well documented. These should be throughly explained to patients who have frequent attacks and who may become dependent or addicted to NSAID medication.

Phenothiazines are an excellent antiemetic in patients who have severe nausea with their attacks. They also have both a pain-relieving and an antidepressant effect. These drugs include, among many, chlorpromazine (Thorazine), which can be administered intramuscularly, rectally, or orally dependent upon the need for rapid effect. All potential side effects of antiemetic drugs must be discussed with the patient.

Preventive Medication

Many medications are used to prevent migraine attacks. These preventive drugs are usually desirable if the recurrence of attacks is significant, the attacks are debilitating, and nondrug treatment is ineffective. Patients having more than four migraine attacks per month merit evaluation for preventive drug programs.

Preventive medications have significant side effects and even adverse results and thus must be carefully monitored and supervised. A preventive program should best be undertaken for a 3- to 6-month period and then discontinued so that the patient's situation can be re-evaluated. Sometimes a natural remission of the migraine occurs and no further medication is required.

Beta blockers are frequently used in preventive programs. Among the present nonselective beta blockers are propranolol (Inderal) and nadolol (Corgard), which block both beta-I and beta-II adrenergic receptors. More selective blockers are metroprolol (Lopressor) and atenolol (Tenormin). Currently there is significant experience and medical literature of beta blocker action in cardiovascular pathology. These beta blockers were initially considered to be effective in migraine because they block the peripheral vasodilatory receptors, but more recently a CNS effect has been postulated.[16]

The dosage must be determined for each individual patient and the patient's cardiovascular status must be determined. Beta blockers cause a lowering of blood pressure and pulse rate (bradycardia), which can be unpleasant and essentially detrimental to the patient. Patients taking beta blockers have experienced confusion and depression, which may negate their value. Cerebrovascular accidents have been attributed to the use of beta blockers, and this devastating complication must always be considered and must be disclosed to the patient.

Recent studies on the relationship of serotonin (5-hydroxytryptamine) and acute ischemic heart disease[17,18] presents an interesting approach that may clarify the relationship of serotonin with migraine and its variants. Serotonin is a vasoactive agent that influences arterial tone during platelet aggregation and deposition. It directly activates serotonergic and alpha-adrenergic receptors by displacing norepinephrine.[19] During platelet aggregation serotonin is released, binding 5-HT receptors that release vasodilating substances. It also binds the 5-HT receptors of the smooth muscles, inducing contraction. In a normal vascular endothelium the response to serotonin is vasodilation. If the endothelium is damaged or in any way impaired the response to serotonin is diminished, with resultant vasoconstriction. How these changes occur in migraine as compared to cardiac ischemia remains problematic, but it is worthy of research, especially because serotonin is a drug related to emotions and vasotonus is related to migraine variants.[20]

Calcium channel blockers are increasingly being evaluated in cardiovascular disease and also in migraine inhibition. The mechanism of calcium blockers remains unknown. Calcium blockers enjoy consideration in patients who have Raynaud's phenomenon or other vasoconstrictive effects from beta blockers, as calcium blockers do not seem to have this effect.

Sansert (methysergide) has been effective in preventing as well as terminating migraine headaches; studies indicate an effectiveness rate of 50 to 80 percent.[16] Its exact mechanism of action remains unknown. Its use is contraindicated in patients with peripheral vascular disease, coronary artery disease, hypertension, pregnancy, and peptic ulcer. The last, peptic ulcer aggravation, is attributed to its enhancement of secretion of gastric acid.[17]

Antidepressants have been advocated and found effective in preventing migraine headaches as well as being antiemetic. Their use has been promoted more in tension headaches than in migraine, but the relationship of tension and migraine (and the accuracy of the term *tension headache*) makes this medication equivocal. Regardless of the etiology of migraine and its relationship to musculoskeletal tension, antidepressants remain a valuable preventive medication; controllable side effects include sedation, dry mouth, and urinary retention.

The recent enthusiasm for Prozac as an antidepressant drug has been encouraging, but its effectiveness as a preventive drug for migraine is limited. Prozac (TCA fluoxetine) is a serotonin-reuptake blocker with minimal anticholinergic effects and weight gain. The severe sequelae recently claimed for a small minority of patients taking Prozac must be borne in mind when prescribing a medication that may require long-term use.

Monoamine oxidase–inhibiting antidepressants (MAOI) have been claimed to be very effective in the prevention of migraine but they must be used judiciously when combined with beta blockers or calcium channel blockers as these latter drugs can cause severe orthostatic hypotension with resultant syncope.

The brain has three classes of 5-HT receptors (5-HT1, 5-HT2, and 5-HT3) which, when stimulated, cause vasoconstriction. As vasodilation is considered pathognomonic of migraine, stimulation of these receptors is therapeutic. Recently, there has been a report of effective treatment of acute migraine by subcutaneous injection of a drug called sumatriptan, which is a specific 5-HT1 agonist.[21] It is a serotonin-like drug without the undesirable side effects and rapid efficacy.

Injection of sumatriptan subcutaneously allegedly provides rapid relief of migraine pain within 10 minutes to 1 hour. Some nausea and photophobia were noted in many patients, but they were considered tolerable, and the patients remained symptom-free for 24 hours. This drug is similar to serotonin but appears to have minimal adverse effects and greater efficacy. It also has fewer side effects than ergotamine and is considered more effective. The medication can be self-administered, after instruction, by the patient.

In summary, any preventive medication program for migraine must be undertaken with care, knowledge of the indications, dosage and contraindication of each drug and careful frequent monitoring for incompatability with other drugs. The organic sequelae in susceptible patients can be ominous and the legal sequelae may also be significant. In the presence of intractable migraine headache, general practitioners should consult with a neurologist who specializes in migraine disorders.

Emergency Room Treatment of Headache

In today's society where a primary physician may not be available, the emergency room has become the site of primary care for many patients. The reasons for a patient resorting to the emergency room are numerous.[22] The patient may be experiencing a headache of unusual severity, resulting in severe anxiety on the part of the patient or the family. A first migraine, one associated with other symptoms, or an unusually prolonged headache that does not respond to medication may also prompt an emergency room visit.

If it is a first headache, other possible organic causes for the headache must be eliminated. This requires a careful history, a thorough neurological and vascular examination, and appropriate neuroimaging procedures, such as spinal tap or CT scan.

If the examination indicates that the headache is the first of a typical migraine or cluster headache, a provocative, diagnostic, and probably therapeutic treatment is justified. The following treatments are suggested:

1. A pain medication such as demerol with an antiemetic
2. Dihydroergotamine with or without an antiemetic[23]
3. Oxygen inhalation
4. Intravenous chlorpromazine[24]
5. Systemic corticosteroids[25]
6. Intravenous prochlorperazine

Careful observation in the ER for an appropriate time is necessary, and follow-up care by the patient's primary physician is mandatory.[26] If there is no primary physician, a return appointment to the emergency room or phone follow-up is imperative until a primary physician assumes care.

REFERENCES

1. Osler, W: The Principles and Practice of Medicine, ed 8. Appleton, New York, 1912, pp 1092–1093.
2. Ad Hoc Committee on Classification of Headache. Arch Neurol 6:173–176, 1963.
3. Dalession, DJ: Pain-sensitive structures within the cranium. In Dalession, DJ (ed): Wolff's Headache and Other Head Pain. Oxford University Press, New York, 1980, pp 24–55.
4. Wolff, HG: Headache and Other Head Pain. Oxford University Press, New York, 1963.
5. Olesen, J, Larsen, B, and Lauritzen, M: Focal hyperemia followed by spreading oligemia and impaired activation of RCBF in classic migraine. Ann Neurol 9:344, 1981.

6. Lashley, KS: Patterns of cerebral integration indicated by the scotomas of migraine. Arch Neurol Psychiatry 46:259–264, 1941.

7. Leao, AAP: Spreading depression of activity in cerebral cortex. J Neurophysiol 7:359–390, 1944.

8. Blau, JN: Premonitory Symptoms of Migraine. In Olesen, L and Edvinsson, L (eds): Basic Mechanisms of Headache. Elsevier, Amsterdam, 1988, pp 345–351.

9. Liveing, E: On Megrim, Sick Headache, and Some Allied Disorders: A Contribution to the Pathology of Nerve Storms. Churchill, London, 1873.

10. Olesen, J: Pathophysiological implications of migraine aura symptomatology. In Olesen, J and Edvinsson, L (eds): Basic Mechanisms of Headache. Elsevier, Amsterdam, 1988, pp 354–363.

10a. Jensen, K, Tfelt-Hansen, P, Lauritzen, M, and Olesen, J: Classic migraine. A prospective recording of symptoms. Acta Neurol Scand 73:359–362, 1986.

10b. Bradshaw, P and Parsons, M: Hemiplegic migraine: A clinical study. Q J Med 34:65–85, 1965.

10c. Bucking, H and Baumgartner, G: Klinik und pathophysiologie der initalen neurologischen symptome bei fokalen migraenen (migraine ophthalmique, migraine accompagne). Arch Psychiatr Nervenkr 219:37–52, 1974.

10d. Peatfield, R: Headache. Springer-Verlag, Berlin, 1986.

11. Turk, DC and Rudy, TE: Neglected topics in the treatment of chronic pain patients—relapse, noncompliance, and adherence enhancement. A Review Article. Pain 44:5–28, 1991.

12. Lipton, SA: Prevention of classic migraine headache by digital massage of the superficial temporal arteries during visual aura. Ann Neurol 19:515–516, 1986.

13. Saper, JR: Headache disorders: Current concepts and treatment strategies. Wright PSG, Littleton, MA, 1983.

14. Rall, TW and Schliefer, LS: In Gilman AG, Goodman, LS, Rall, TW, and Murad, F (eds): Pharmacological Basis of Therapeutics, ed 7. Macmillan, New York, 1985, pp 926–945.

15. Saper, JR, and Jones, JM: Ergotamine tartrate dependency: features and possible mechanisms. Clin Neuropharm 9:244–256, 1986.

16. Lance, JW: Mechanism and Management of Headache, ed 4. Butterworth Scientific, London, 1982.

17. Saper, JR: Headache Disorders: Current Concepts and Treatment Strategies. Wright PSG, Littleton, MA, 1983.

18. Hillis, LD and Lange, RA: Serotonin and acute ischemic heart disease. New Engl J Med 324:688–689, 1991.

19. Peatfield, RC, Fozard, JR, and Rose, FC: Drug treatment of migraine. In Rose, FC (ed): Handbook of Clinical Neurology, Vol 48. Elsevier, Amsterdam, 1986, pp 173–216.

20. Vanmhoutte, PM, Cohen, RA, and Van Neueten, JM: Serotonin and arterial vessels. J Cardiovasc Pharmacol 6 (Suppl 2):S421–S428, 1984.

21. Cady, RK, Wendt, JK, Kirchner, JR, Sargent, JD, Rothrock, JF, and Skaggs, H.: Treatment of acute migraine with subcutaneous sumatriptan. JAMA 265(21):2831–2835, 1991.

22. Edmeads, J: Emergency room management of headache. Headache 28:675–679, 1988.

23. Callahan, M and Raskin, NH: A controlled study of dihydroergotamine in the treatment of acute migraine headache. Headache 26:168–171, 1986.

24. Lane, PL and Ross, R: Intravenous chlropromazine—preliminary results in acute migraine. Headache 25:302–304, 1985.

25. Gallagher, RM: Emergency treatment of intractable migraine. Headache 25:164, 1985.

26. Dickman, RL and Master, T: The management of nontraumatic headache in a university hospital emergency room. Headache 19:391–396, 1979.

CHAPTER 3

Cluster Headaches and Variants

The cluster headache has the reputation of being the most severe epidemic form of headache known to humanity. It has several terminologies: red migraine, erythromelalgia, sphenopalatine neuralgia,[1] hemicrania periodica neuralgiformis, periodic migrainous neuralgia,[2] and ciliary neuralgia.[3] Because it could be initiated by a histamine provocation test, it was termed "histaminic headache."[4] The term "cluster headache" has been formally recognized by the Ad Hoc Committee on the Classification of Headache[5] and more recently by the Headache Classification Committee of the International Headache Society.[6]

CLINICAL FEATURES OF CLUSTER HEADACHE

In contrast to classical migraine, cluster headaches occur primarily in males at a ratio of 4–6:1. The onset is typically in the late twenties, but onset has been reported in children as young as 1 year and persons as old as 70 years.

In its classic form, the headaches come in clusters, one or two per year, each lasting for about 2 to 3 months. Periodicity is the most striking characteristic of cluster headaches. The periods of duration and occurrence of the clusters are consistent for a given person. A seasonal aspect for cluster headache has not been verified.[7] Table 3–1 shows the classification of cluster headache used by the International Headache Society.

Cluster headaches have no aura, either visual or neurological, and no prodrome. The headache begins abruptly and builds up to a climax in 10 to

Table 3–1. INTERNATIONAL HEADACHE SOCIETY CLASSIFICATION OF CLUSTER HEADACHE

3.1 Cluster headache
    3.1.1. Cluster headache periodicity undetermined
    3.1.2. Episodic cluster headache
    3.1.3. Chronic cluster headache
        3.1.3.1 Chronic cluster headache unremitting from onset
        3.1.3.2 Chronic cluster headache evolved from episodic
3.2 Chronic paroxysmal hemicrania
3.3 Chronic clusterlike disorder not fulfilling above criteria

15 minutes. The typical cluster headache is unilateral, but it may change sides from one attack to another.

Pain is usually distributed through the first and second division of the trigeminal nerve, especially the orbital, retro-orbital, temporal, supraorbital, and infraorbital areas. The frequency of the site decreases in that sequence.[8]

One-fifth of patients complain of severe pain in extratrigeminal regions such as the back of the neck, the suboccipital region, and the carotid artery region of the front of the neck.

The pain is described by the patient as "excruciating"; it may be characterized as a boring (in) but, unlike migraine, it is rarely termed "throbbing." The pain usually lasts 45 minutes to 1 hour. Often the patient states that it feels like the eyeball is being pushed out of its socket.

The attacks have a striking regularity, and for that reason they have been termed "circadian."[9] The patient may have an attack at the same time of day every day for a number of weeks. Nocturnal attacks are experienced in 50 percent of patients with the same periodicity. Sleep studies have determined that these occur during both REM and non-REM periods.[10,11]

Besides the severe pain, there are other symptoms attributable to overactivity of the parasympathetic nervous system: ipsilateral lacrimation (eye tearing), conjunctival injection, and nasal stuffiness. A minor Horner's syndrome can be observed. Facial flushing and/or pallor with facial and scalp tenderness or paresthesia has been noted. Bradycardia is frequently also noted.[12]

Whereas the typical migraine headache patient seeks solitude and quiet darkness during an attack, the patient with cluster headache is usually restless and unable to sit quietly. If the patient does assume a rest position, it is usually sitting with the head down and held firmly between the hands. It is not infrequent that the patient cries or screams out during an attack. Many patients exhibit anxiety by pacing, jumping, or even running during an attack; this gives an indication of the severity of the pain.

Personality studies have been performed in an attempt to determine the personality type that is prone to cluster headache. A "leonine-mouse" facial appearance has been described,[13] but there appears to be no typical appearance.

Fully 80 percent of patients are heavy smokers and have a history of excessive use of alcohol. Patients generally avoided alcohol during an attack, however, as alcohol consumption aggravates an attack because of its vasodilatory effect. Many cluster headache patients have been described as ambitious, proficient, goal-oriented, compulsive, but insecure: a typical type A personality.[14] This personality type together with the potential for substance abuse and addiction to medication—ergotamine, analgesics, etc.—makes treatment of these patients difficult.

There is a high incidence of gastric ulcer in these patients[15] as well as proneness to hypertension and coronary heart disease. This increases the possibility of adverse interactions between various prescribed medications. Alcohol may precipitate an attack, as may the use of nitroglycerin for angina or histaminelike medications for upper respiratory infections. An astute and careful evaluation of the patient and the proffered treatment is mandatory in caring for these patients, as is a determination of patient compliance with the treatment program.

CLUSTER HEADACHE VARIANTS

For a specific diagnosis of classic cluster headache the episodes (1) must occur for periods lasting 7 days to 1 year, and (2) be separated by pain-free periods of time lasting 14 or more days. There are many variants of the cluster headache disorder that warrant discussion.

1. *Cluster-tic syndrome.* Cluster headache occurs in conjunction with a trigeminal neuralgia *(tic douloureax).*

2. *Cluster-vertigo.* Vertigo occurs during a cluster headache but not during a remission.[16]

3. *Cluster-migraine.* Cluster headache occurs in a patient with an established migraine headache history. In these cases an aura may precede the migraine but not the cluster headache. It is possible to distinguish readily between the two types of headache experienced by the individual.[17] This relationship of cluster and migraine occurs in 1 to 3 percent of either patient population.[18]

4. *Cluster-like headache with organic lesions.* Cluster headaches have been associated with intracranial vascular and space-occupying lesions such as meningiomas, pituitary adenoma, and arteriovenous malformations.[19]

5. *Cluster-like headache after head or face trauma.* The relationship between the trauma and the cluster headache is unclear.[20]

6. *After infections.* It is apparent that diagnosing a cluster headache

requires a search for associated syndromes especially when the results of treatment and follow-up observation are atypical.

PATHOPHYSIOLOGY OF CLUSTER HEADACHE

Areas of ischemia of the involved supraorbital area, depicted by thermography have been reported and assumed to be pathognomonic of cluster headaches.[21] The fact that cluster headaches can be precipitated by the ingestion of alcohol, histamine, and nitroglycerin—all vasodilators—implies vasodilation as the etiological basis of this headache. Enhanced pulsations of the intraocular bed occur during cluster headaches but have not been observed during migraine.[22] Regional cerebral blood flow studies, however, have not confirmed these findings.[23]

An increase in temporal artery pulsations is associated with cluster headache, indicating an increase in extracranial blood flow following the onset of pain. This suggests a primary neurological rather than a primary vascular etiology. As there is agreement that there is extracranial vasodilation in cluster headaches secondary to neuronal discharge through the trigeminal nerve, central mechanisms are postulated. The hypothalamus regulates the autonomic nervous system and is also considered the base for circadian periodicity, which is so characteristic of cluster headache.

As the nerve distribution of a cluster headache is in the distribution of the first and second divisions of the trigeminal nerve, studies have ensued to determine this relationship. The vascular system of the trigeminal nerve has been implicated.[24] Also, patients with intractable cluster headaches have derived benefit from destructive lesions of the trigeminal nerve.

The hypothalamus may be involved in cluster headaches. It regulates the autonomic system and is, with the suprachiasmic nuclei, possibly the base of circadian periodicity.[25] The sleep cycle, which is also impaired in many cluster headache patients, is possibly located here. The therapeutic significance of this central mechanism remains conjectural, but with further study greater pharmacological management of serotonin may be beneficial. Serotonin has been found to be elevated in cluster headaches and has a relationship to the neurochemical aspects of the central autonomic nervous system.[26]

There are well-documented brain stem connections between the periaqueductal gray matter, the midbrain dorsal raphe nuclei, the reticular formation, and the nuclei of the trigeminal nerve. These may be the neural links between the hypothalamus and the trigeminal nerve in the evolution of cluster headache.

The neurological aspects of the cluster headache incriminate the autonomic and parasympathetic nervous systems, as is manifested by the presence of a Horner's syndrome (sympathetic), forehead and facial sweating, lacrimation, nasal congestion, hypotension, and bradycardia (parasympathetic nervous system) in cluster headache patients. The site of this neurological impairment is postulated to be a pathological focus located in the superior pericarotid cavernous sinus plexus, which is where the fibers from the ophthalmic trigeminal division, the maxillary division, and the superior cervical ganglion join together (see Fig. 1–1).[27] At this site there is a convergence of afferent (sensory) and autonomic fibers.

As can be seen in Fig. 1–1, the numerous branches from this plexus supply all the regions that are involved in the cluster headache:[28]

1. The branches from the ophthalmic division to the circle of Willis
2. The maxillary branches to the orbital ciliary nerve
3. The orbital ciliary nerve, which supplies sensory branches to the orbit
4. The sympathetic branches, which supply the carotid artery

A lesion at the cavernous sinus plexus could elicit all the components of the cluster headache. Because the sphenopalatine ganglion is included in these nervous pathways, a sphenopalatine nerve block may be considered to alleviate the cluster symptoms.

The cause of cluster headache currently can be summarized as being neuronal discharges within the branches of the trigeminal nerve originating from the circadian center at the thalamic level. The symptoms are mediated ultimately via vasomotor dilatory effects.

MANAGEMENT OF CLUSTER HEADACHES

The pharmacological treatment of cluster headache is very similar to the acute treatment of migraine headache, but there are significant differences. The symptoms of the typical cluster headache are so severe that after cessation of the acute attack, the patient lives in fear of a recurrence, especially if he or she knows about the natural periodicity of cluster headache.

There are some preventive measures of value, but none that are as promising or effective as those advised for prevention of migraine. Developing a treatment protocol that assures the patient possible and immediate relief is the most reassuring aspect of preventive treatment.

Many patients are type A personalities, heavy smokers, and heavy alcohol consumers, and these lifestyles all provoke cluster headaches. Unfortunately, current medical expertise experiences failure in remedying or modifying these behavioral patterns.

Fear of recurrences of cluster headaches has actually promoted severe depression and even contemplation of suicide. These psychological features benefit from psychotherapeutic measures and even antidepressant drugs, but the latter have certain contraindications and complications. Pharmacological prophylaxis will be discussed in details later in this chapter.

As the attack is abrupt and crescendos within 10 to 15 minutes and lasts 45 minutes, immediate treatment is indicated and should be readily available. The following have been found useful and effective.

Oxygen Inhalation

Oxygen administered through a face mask at the rate of 8 liters per minute for 10 minutes may abort or significantly minimize a cluster headache.[29] Inhalation must be initiated at the very beginning of the headache, so the oxygen equipment must literally be carried by the patient for immediate use. A delay may result in a recurrence shortly after the delayed attempt at aborting an attack; the headache then persists in spite of reuse of oxygen. A small canister of oxygen attached to a mask can easily be carried in a briefcase or be available in the usual sites of daily activities: the office, the home, the bedside, and in the car.

As attacks tend to occur after an infection or minor head trauma, these should alert the patient and ensure that all treatment modalities be available at that time.

The benefit of oxygen in cluster headache suggests that vasodilation is causative, as oxygen is known to normally produce cerebral vasoconstriction. During an attack of cluster headache cerebrovascular circulation has been shown to have an abnormal reaction to oxygen, which is apparently corrected by increased oxygenation.[30] Between attacks the cerebrovascular circulation response to oxygen remains normal, indicating that the episodic abnormal responsiveness to oxygen during an attack is remedied by inhalation of O^2. Oxygen also stimulates synthesis of serotonin, which has been found to be diminished in cluster headache.[31]

Ergotamine

Because cluster headaches have such an abrupt onset and crescendo, any medication must be administered in a manner that is rapidly absorbed to be effective. In cluster headaches it is known that there is a gastroparesis (diminished gastric mobility and absorption), so oral medications are poorly absorbed and thus are ineffective in aborting a cluster headache.[32]

Ergotamine suppositories are effective, but cluster headache patients are usually irritable, hyperactive, and unable to remain still; thus suppositories are not inserted and retained adequately to be effective.

Ergotamine inhalation (Medihaler Ergotamine-Riker) has proven to be effective when used within the first 5 minutes of an attack. This means of administration has proven more effective than oral tablets or suppositories, exceeded only in effectiveness by intravenous ergotamine.[33]

Ergotamine inhalation must be carefully monitored to ensure an adequate plasma concentration. As many as six inhalations may be needed. The spray (as delivered by the current method) has its major effect upon the mucosa of the bronchial tree and may not deliver an adequate dosage to the blood plasma. For inhalation to be effective the patient must practice and determine the most effective manner to use the inhalant.

Sublingual ergotamine is the next most effective method of delivery. This sublingual medication must also be administered early in an attack to be effective.

Ergotamine remains the most effective medication in the treatment of cluster headache. With sublingual delivery it is effective in 35 percent of patients within 4 to 9 minutes and in 65 percent of patients within 10 to 15 minutes.[33] As cluster headaches last for only 15 to 45 minutes, these statistics are difficult to put into perspective. It is possible that ergotamine (and oxygen) merely delay the headache attack but the severity may persist and cause the patient to repeat the medication. This may result in drug habituation and abuse.

The side effects of ergotamine include nausea, vomiting, extremity paresthesia, leg muscle cramps, and the more ominous coronary artery spasm with angina. There may also be mental cloudiness and confusion, and the peripheral vasoconstrictive effects and peripheral neuropathy may persist. All these side effects must be taken into consideration when ergotamine is prescribed.

Dihydroergotamine

Dihydroergotamine (DHE) has become available in an injectable form for rapid absorption. This medication is available in an intramuscular as well as intravenous application and if the patient or a member of the family can be adequately trained for proper administration, this means affords more rapid relief of a cluster headache. The pharmacology of DHE is identical to ergotamine, as are the side effects. Overuse of DHE is a cause for concern: when pain relief is insufficient, the patient may reinject and set up a cycle of overuse.

The mechanism by which ergotamine or dihydroergotamine works remains obscure, but recent studies using radioactive ergotamine (3hDHE) reveals a bonding site in the midbrain nuclei. This seems to confirm the probability that ergotamine acts via a central mechanism.

Local Anesthetic Agents

Anesthetic agents locally applied to the nasal mucosa and to the sphenopalatine nucleus have proven effective. Lidocaine nasal drops fall into this category.[34] With the patient in a supine position and the head turned to the side of the headache, Lidocaine drops (1 cc of a 2% solution) are applied through a nose dropper. These drops may be repeated twice at 15-minute intervals and have proven effective in a number of patients.

A local application of cocaine on a cotton applicator to the middle turbinates was advocated in the past, but is no longer available because of the fear of addiction. A 10% cocaine solution was also advocated but is no longer, for the same reasons.[35]

Steroids

Although steroids are advocated in prophylactic treatment of cluster headaches, their use in an acute attack may be dramatic. Reportedly, 30 mgm of prednisone given IM has reportedly given prompt relief that may last for 10 or more days.[36] The side effects of steroids must be judiciously considered in using this medication for repeated acute attacks.

Analgesics and Narcotics

Many patients with cluster headache have significant residual head pain for which they require analgesics and even narcotics to attain acceptable relief. Benefit from oral analgesics and mild narcotics is questioned as being a placebo effect because of the gastroparesis and poor absorption known to occur in cluster headache. Usually, the classic cluster headache subsides in 45 minutes and further medication should be discouraged.

PROPHYLAXIS OF CLUSTER HEADACHES

Preventive management of the frightening and excruciating aspect of cluster headaches has obviously been strongly requested by patients and attempted by their physicians. As the preventive aspects used with migraine headaches are not as effective in cluster headache, a pharmacological prophylaxis is usually advocated.

Prophylaxis consists of initiating the proffered medication early in the cluster cycle and continuing the medication daily until the patient is free of symptoms for at least 2 weeks. Medication then is best gradually decreased rather than abruptly terminated. The same medication that has proven effective may then be restarted at the onset of the next cluster.

There are a number of beneficial prophylactic medications of proven value: ergotamine, methysergide, corticosteroids, lithium carbonate, calcium blockers, and indomethacin. Other medications have proven less beneficial: chlorpromazine, beta blockers, tricyclic antidepressants, and phenylpropanolamine. Histamine desensitization has also been disappointing.

As most cluster headaches are abrupt in onset and of limited duration, the effectiveness of prophylactic medication is difficult to evaluate. Such medication may not fully abort that attack but rather merely delay its crescendo. In patients who undergo numerous attacks in a single day, there can be a tendency to overmedicate in anticipation of the expected number. Overmedication is understandable as it is well-documented that if a cluster is not aborted early or effectively there may be residual pain and suffering for months. The patient who has experienced this may, understandably, overreact by taking excessive prophylactic medication.

As all attacks may not be eliminated or prevented but merely diminished in severity and frequency, the doctor must weigh the benefits against the possibility of overmedication, undesirable side effects, and/or rebound. A good patient-doctor relationship is necessary in determining the proper prophylactic program. Every clinic specializing in the treatment of migraine, migraine variant, and cluster headache has a precise protocol, but each must be equated with a specific patient, the precise type of headache, and reaction to medications, as well as ancillary medical problems requiring medication.

Ergotamine Used Prophylactically

Ergotamine 1 mgm taken orally twice daily has proven effective, but in this case, ergotamine should not be used to abort an acute attack.[37] An acute episode should be treated by oxygen inhalation.[38] Ergotamine can be combined with corticosteroids, lithium, or verapamil. A nocturnal dose of oral ergotamine (one of the recommended b.i.d.) should be given to prevent a nocturnal attack. In the event of chronic cluster headache, habituation of ergotamine must be carefully evaluated.

Dihydroergotamine

In patients who experience repeated cluster attacks, the use of intravenous dihydroergotamine (DHE) given in 8-hour sequence for 72 hours may break the cycle and cause a remission.

Corticosteroids

Reports on the efficacy of steroids in prevention of cluster attacks has been promising. A course of prednisone 40 mgm daily for 2 weeks has been advocated, then tapered down in 1 week.[36] Recurrence of headache after discontinuation mandates the use of a different medication. If prednisone is not effective in 48 to 72 hours, another drug should be considered. The undesirable side effects of prolonged steroid use must be kept in mind.

Lithium

Lithium, well documented as an antidepressant medication, has also been found effective in the prophylaxis of cluster headaches.[39] Lithium is not a sedative or depressant, but it is a mood stabilizer. It reduces the sleep REM period in depressed patients, which may be a factor in its efficacy in cluster headache patients as cluster headaches have been related to REM sleep.[40] Although the precise mechanism of lithium remains obscure, it is known that lithium has no effect upon cerebral hemodynamics.[41]

The recommended daily dose is 600 to 900 mgm, which is a lesser dosage than that used in manic depressive psychosis. Benefit should manifest itself within 1 week if lithium is to be effective. Even patients who benefit from lithium (40 percent) also require intermittent ergotamine therapy. After several months on lithium the benefit wanes; patients become refractory to further lithium and must revert to another medication.

There are side effects of lithium that may neutralize its benefit. These are tremor, slurred speech, lethargy, confusion, seizures, and extrapyramidal (parkinsonism type) symptoms.

Calcium Channel Blockers

Calcium channel blockers have evoked a flurry of interest in the treatment of vascular headaches, especially migraine and variants. Their use in cluster headaches has also been advocated.[42] Verapamil has been considered the most effective in doses of 120 mgm three to four times daily. Calcium blockers can be combined with ergotamine or lithium. Several blockers such as Nifedipine, Nomodipine, and Diltiazem have had their exponents. Nifedipine is effective but causes a headache per se that disappoints patients.

The undesirable side effects of calcium blockers include constipation, water retention, and weight gain, but all these are accepted if the blockers are effective against the headaches.

Indomethacin

This nonsteroidal anti-inflammatory agent (NSAID) has been extremely effective therapeutically usually within 48 hours of ingestion and is even used as a diagnostic agent to confirm the diagnosis early in the disease. Indomethacin is most effective in short-duration "sharp" headaches of abrupt onset. The major contraindication is gastric irritation, and there have been occasional complaints of confusion. Taking the drug with meals and with an antacid usually prevents the gastric symptoms.

Histamine Desensitization

Histamine desensitization was advised as a preventive for cluster headaches when the etiology of these headaches was considered to be a histamine reaction. Histamine subcutaneously administered had been in vogue to prophylactically treat cluster headaches, but the attempt at sensitization became increasingly difficult and ineffectual, so it now is rarely used.[43]

Beta Blockers

Beta blockers, though effective in migraine headaches, have not been significantly valuable in cluster prophylactic treatment. The usual bradycardia noted during a cluster episode presents a complication to using these blockers to prevent a cluster.

Occipital Nerve Block

As the manifestations of cluster headaches are often in the greater superior occipital nerve distribution, a nerve block of this area has proven effective. It is postulated that there is a decrease of afferent input to the trigeminal nerve via the C-2 branch and the spinal tract and nucleus of the Vth nerve, and not merely blocking the dermatome of the nerve as the basis of the injection. Remissions of 5 to 70 days have been reported, but only if steroids are added to the anesthetic agent injected.[44]

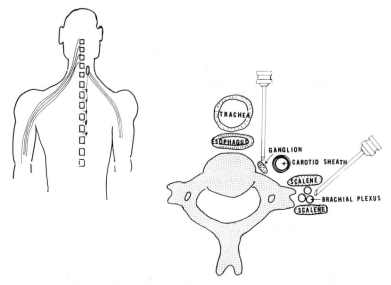

Figure 3–1. Technique of stellate ganglion sympathetic chemical block.
Depicts the area of injecting the stellate ganglion and the vital structures in its vicinity. The brachial plexus block is also shown but is rarely needed in head and face pain.

SURGICAL TREATMENT OF
INTRACTABLE CLUSTER HEADACHES

There have been several surgical procedures advocated in intractable cluster headache, including interruption of the sympathetic nerve supply and the trigeminal nerve.

The former indicates interruption of the sympathetic system by stellate chemical blocks (Fig. 3–1). Trigeminal nerve gangliorhizolysis by per cutaneous radio frequency requires consultation by a trained anesthesiologist.[45] For this procedure to be invoked, the cluster headache must be consistently on the same unilateral side, there must be a total failure to respond to medical treatment, and the patient must have a stable personality that can accept the residual loss of sensation.[46]

In summary, it can be stated that the treatment of the cluster headache patient requires a close patient-physician relationship with an interested and knowledgeable physician who will carefully and consistently monitor the patient's reaction to medication, tolerance of side effects, psychological acceptance of the disease, and willingness to adhere to and comply with the recommended procedures.

REFERENCES

1. Sluder, RG: The syndrome of sphenopalatine ganglion neurosis. Am J Med Sci 140:868, 1910.
2. Harris, W: Neuritis and Neuralgia. Oxford University Press, London, 1926, p 918.
3. Harris, W: Ciliary migrainous neuralgia and its treatment. Brit Med J 1:457–460, 1936.
4. Horton, BT, Maclean, AR, and Craig, WM: A new syndrome of vascular headache results in treatment with histamine: Preliminary report. Mayo Clin Proc 14:257–260, 1939.
5. Ad Hoc Committee on Classification of Headache. JAMA 179:717–718, 1962.
6. Headache Classification Committee of International Headache Society: Classification and diagnostic criteria for headache disorders, cranial neuralgia, and facial pain. Cephalalgia 8 (Suppl 7):1–96, 1988.
7. Kudrow, L.: Migraine: Clinical and research aspects. In Blau, JN (ed), Johns Hopkins, Baltimore, 1987, pp 113–133.
8. Manzoni, GL, Terano, MG, Bono, G, Micieli G, Martucci N, and Nappi, G: Cluster headache: Clinical findings in 180 patients. Cephalalgia 3:21–30, 1983.
9. Ekbom, K.: Pattern of cluster headaches with a note on the relation to angina pectoris and peptic ulcer. Acta Neurol Scand 46:225–237, 1970.
10. Kudrow, L., McGinty, DJ, Phillips, ER, and Stevenson, M: Sleep apnea in cluster headache. Cephalalgia 4:33–38, 1984.
11. Mathew, NT, Glaze, D, and Frost, J: Sleep apnea and other sleep abnormalities in primary headache disorders. In Rose, C (ed): Migraine Proceedings. Fifth International Migraine Symposium, London (1989), pp 40–49 (Krager) Basel (1985).
12. Bruyn, GW, Bootsma, BK, and Klawans, HL: Cluster headache and bradycardia. Headache 16:11–15, 1976.
13. Graham, JR: Cluster headache. Headache 11:175–185, 1972.
14. Friedman, AP and Mikropoulos, HE: Cluster headache. Neur 8:653–666, 1958.
15. Kudrow, L: Prevalence of migraine, peptic ulcer, coronary heart disease, and hypertension in cluster headache. Headache 16:66–69, 1976.
16. Gilbert, GJ: Meniere's syndrome and cluster headache: Recurrent paroxysmal focal vasodilatation. JAMA 11:691–694, 1965.
17. Medina, JL and Diamond, S: The clinical link between migraine and cluster headache. Arch Neurol 34:470–472, 1977.
18. Solomon, S, Kartunkel, P, and Guglielmo, KM: Migraine-cluster headache syndrome. Headache 25:236–239, 1985.
19. Mani, S and Deeter, J: Arteriovenous malformation of the brain presenting as cluster headache—a case report. Headache 22:184–185, 1982.
20. Mathew, NT and Rueveni, U: Cluster-like headache following trauma. Headache 28:297, 1988.
21. Friedman, AP and Wood, EH: Thermography in vascular headache. In Uema, S (ed): Medical Thermography. Brentwood Publishers, Los Angeles, 1976, pp 80–84.
22. Horven, I, Nornes, H, and Sjaastad, O: Different corneal indentation pulse patterns in cluster headaches and migraine. Neurol 22:92–98, 1972.
23. Norris, JW, Hachinski, VC, and Cooper, PW: Cerebral blood flow changes in cluster headache. Acta Neurol Scand 54:371–374, 1976.
24. Moskowitz, MA: Neurobiology of vascular head pain. J Ann Neurol 16:157–168, 1984.
25. Kudrow, L: The cyclic relationship of natural illumination to cluster period frequency. Cepalalgia 7 (Suppl 6):76–78, 1987.
26. Groos, G, Mason, R, and Meijer, J: Electrical and pharmacological properties of the suprachiasmic nuclei. Fed Proc 42:2790–2795, 1983.
27. Moskowitz, MA: Neurobiology of vascular head pain. J Ann Neurol 16:157–168, 1984.

28. Dalessio, DJ: Pain-sensitive structures within the cranium. In Dalessio, DJ (ed): Wolff's Headache and Other Head Pain, ed 4. Oxford University Press, Oxford, 1980, pp 24–55.
29. Kudrow, L: Response of cluster headache attacks to oxygen inhalation. Headache 21:1–4, 1981.
30. Sakai, F and Meyer, JS: Abnormal cerebrovascular reactivity in patients with migraine and cluster headache. Headache 19:257–266, 1979.
31. Costa, E and Meek, JL: Regulation of the biosynthesis of catecholamines and serotonin in the CNS. Ann Rev Pharmacol 14:491–511, 1974.
32. Kudrow, L: Cluster Headache: Mechanism and Management. Oxford University Press, Oxford, 1980.
33. Ekbom, K, Paalzow, L, Tfelt-Hansen, P, and Walenlind, E: Optional routes of administration of ergotamine tartrate in cluster headache patients: A pharmaceutical study. Cephalalgia 3:15–20, 1983.
34. Kitelle, JP, Grouse, DS, and Seybord, ME: Cluster headache: Local anaesthetic abortive agents. Arch Neurol 42:496–498, 1985.
35. Barre, F: Cocaine as an abortive agent to cluster headache. Headache 22:69–73, 1982.
36. James, JL: The treatment of cluster headaches with prednisone. Dis Nerv Syst 36:275–376, 1975.
37. Ekbom, KA: Ergotamine tartrate orally: Histaminic Cephalalgia, Horton, Harris, Ciliary Neuralgia. Acta Psychiat Scan 46:106–113, 1947.
38. Mathew, NT: Cluster Headache and Variants. Presented at Meeting of the American Association for the Study of Headache, Scottsdale, AZ, January 24–26, 1991.
39. Mathew, NT: Clinical subtypes of cluster headaches and response to lithium therapy. Headache 18:26–30, 1978.
40. Mendels, J, and Chernik, DA: The effect of lithium carbonate on the sleep of depressed patients. Int Pharmaco-Psychiat 8:184–192, 1973.
41. Okayasu, H, Meyer, JS, Mathew, NT, et al: Lithium carbonate has no measurable effect on cerebral hemodynamics in cluster headaches. Headache 24:1–4, 1984.
42. Meyer, JS and Harendberg, J: Clinical effectiveness of calcium entry blockers in prophylactic treatment of migraine and cluster headaches. Headache 23:266–277, 1983.
43. Campbell, JK: The Current Status of Histamine Desensitization in the Treatment of Cluster Headache. Spectrum Publications, New York, 1984, pp 111–118.
44. Anthony, M: Arrest of Attacks of Cluster Headache by Local Steroid Injection of the Occipital Nerve. In Rose, FC (ed): Migraine: Clinical and Research Advances. Karger, Basel, 1985, pp 169–173.
45. Onofrio, BM and Campbell, JK: Surgical treatment of chronic cluster headache. Mayo Clin Proc 61:537–544, 1986.
46. Ekbom, K, Lindgren, L, Nilsson, BY, Hardebo, JE, and Waldenlind, E: Retro-gasserian glycerol injection in the treatment of chronic cluster headache. Cephalalgia 7:21–27, 1987.

CHAPTER 4

The Common Daily Headache

Volumes have been written in the medical literature about both the migraine headache and the cluster headache. These headaches are severe and pleasure-threatening to the sufferer, but they represent only a small portion of the headache complaints that confront the physician almost daily.

Almost three out of four American adults (73 percent) studied in a 1985 survey suffered one or more headaches in a year.[1] Headache patients were considered more troublesome than low-back-pain patients. Headaches prevent a large number of employees from functioning. An estimated 4 billion sick days were lost by all adults in 1985 (approximately 23 days per person per year); undoubtedly a large percentage of these were headache patients.[1]

Patients who suffer with headache vary in all age groups, but there are fewer with increasing age. Women suffer from headaches more than men, and whites more than blacks. College graduates report more headaches than do high school graduates, and those in higher income brackets more than those in the lowest bracket. Homemakers were found to have the same incidence as professional or skilled laborers.[1] This tends to belie the view that professional or skilled workers experience more stress than housewives.

The Hassle scale measures "the irritating, frustrating, distressing demands that to some degree characterize everyday transactions with the environment."[2] The scale is based on the degree to which these demands impair the individual's physical and emotional health. Fully 82 percent of high scorers suffer from headache, as compared to 67 percent with backache complaints.

The types of daily and/or chronic headaches are numerous, including muscular and vascular tension headaches, paranasal sinus headaches, and headaches termed ocular, dental, otalgic (ear pain), posttraumatic, TMJ, neurological, and neurosurgical. Many of these types are of sufficient significance to warrant a full chapter in this book. Tables 4–1 and 4–2 list types

53

Table 4–1. PARTIAL LIST OF CAUSES
OF HEADACHES

Intracranial Causes

A. Toxic
   Carbon monoxide
   Toxic fumes
   Side effects of drugs: NSAIDs,
      antihypertensive, etc.
   Heavy metals
   Withdrawal headache from habit-
      ual uses
B. Metabolic
   Febrile illness
   Hepatic disease
   Renal disease
   Endocrine imbalance
   Cushing's disease
   Hypoparathyroidism
   Postseizure headache
   Hypo- and hyperthyroid disease
C. Infectious Diseases
   1. Meningeal acute bacterial men-
         ingitis
      Acute viral meningitis
      Spirochetal meningitis (syphi-
         lis, etc.)
   2. Parenchymal
      Syphilis
      Viral encephalitis (chronic)
      Viral encephalitis (acute)
      Toxoplasma

Extracranial Causes

A. Infectious
   Sinusitis
   Mastoiditis } bacterial, fungal, etc.
   Tonsillitis
   Herpetic
B. Vascular
   Vasculitis
   Carotid dissection
   Carotid occlusion (thrombus)
   Paget's disease

C. Dental
   Pulpitis
   Periodontitis
   Dentinal
   Cemental
   Odontalgia (atypical)
D. Bone and Joint
   Temporomandibular
   Osteomyelitis
   Eagle's syndrome
   Metastasis (skull)
E. Tumor
   Carcinoma
   Lymphoepithelioma
F. Cranial Neuralgias
   Trigeminal neuralgia
   Glossopharyngeal neuroma
   Occipital neuralgia
   Atypical facial pain
G. Vascular
   Temporal arteritis
   Stroke TIA
   Infectious vasculitis (herpes zos-
      ter, simplex, etc.)
   Granulomatous arteritis
H. Increased Intracranial Pressure
   Tumor
   Abscess
   Hematoma (subdural, epidural,
      parenchymal, etc.)
I. Decreased Intracranial Pressure
   CFS leak: postspinal tap
J. Tumor Invasion of Peripheral Nerves
K. Posttrauma Headache
   Postconcussion

Table 4–2. FUNCTIONAL IDEOPATHIC HEADACHES

I. Vascular Headache
   A. Migraine
   B. Migraine variant
   C. Exertional headache
   D. Postcoital headache
   E. Post–cold ingestion headache (ice cream)

II. Cluster Headache
   A. Acute cyclical cluster headache
   B. Chronic cluster headache
   C. Cluster headache variants
      1. Cluster migraine
      2. Chronic paroxysmal hemicrania

III. Cervicogenic Headache (of questionable etiology; see Chapter 5)

IV. Tension Headache

V. Chronic Daily Headache (ideopathic or of numerous etiologies)

of headache according to numerous etiologies. The lists are by no means exhaustive.

A recent study of 22,071 U.S. male physicians aged 40 to 80 years showed that they ingested 325 mgm/d aspirin. This allegedly produced a 20 percent reduction in the recurrence rate of migraine.[3] The study concluded that aspirin is analgesic and anti-inflammatory. Aspirin also inhibits platelet aggregation which contains serotonin and thus indicates a possible mechanism for migrainelike headache.[4] A recent double-blind study of nonmigrainous headache patients revealed that caffeine alone was as effective in relieving headache as the combination of caffeine and a mild analgesic such as acetaminophen.[5]

The vascular component of many headaches is also a factor. Vascular dilatation per se is not painful, but edema from dilatation may be painful even though edema does not necessarily indicate increased blood flow. How these peripheral factors interact or create central neuronal activity remains unclear. Treatment of "vascular" (or neurogenic) headache therefore remains empirical yet effective. In time we may understand why such treatment is effective.

The symptom of headache presents a significant psychosocial dilemma.[6] There are many psychophysiological and/or behavioral factors related to headaches. The patient experiencing head pain may conjure up images of brain tumors, stroke, and severe organic disease. These fears must be addressed.

Terms such as "migraine personality" and "headache personality type" are unhelpful because they suggest that the patient's suffering is "all in the mind." But this psychological assessment does not mitigate the patient's pain. People with severe, recurrent, and persistent headache are disabled, aggitated, and in need of consideration and assistance. (The psychological aspects of head and face pain will be discussed in Chapter 10.)

A number of factors have been claimed to precipitate headache, including stress, menses, specific food substances, the weather, trauma, various allergies, fumes, bright lights, physical exercise, and specific movements of the head and neck. It becomes obvious that there is no common denominator. The traditional concepts regarding the mechanisms, etiology, and exact neurovascular aspects of headache are being constantly reviewed in view of the controversies surrounding diagnosis and accepted treatments. Many intermittent headaches gradually progress to become chronic daily headaches. This suggests a central neurological mechanism, which may become the basis for the management of headaches.

The precipitating factors listed above are not all amenable to medication, change in daily activities, emotional reaction, or general physical conditioning. However, where possible, these factors should be manipulated or modified in hope that relief will result.

The severity of the headache may simplistically be quantified as

1. *Disabling*
2. *Severe:* activities limited 50 to 90 percent of normal
3. *Moderate:* activities limited 25 to 50 percent of normal
4. *Mild:* activities not limited in any measurable degree

This qualification is highly subjective as the "normal" activities curtailed cannot be standardized.

TENSION HEADACHE

A most commonly diagnosed headache of limited or unrevealed organic etiology has been termed "tension headache," implying that the head pain is the result of unrelenting muscular contraction. The basis for this sustained muscular tension remains obscure, with psychological causation being considered the predominant factor.

Tension headache is defined by the Ad Hoc Committee on Classification of Headache as an "ache or sensation of tightness, pressure, or constriction, widely varied in intensity, frequency, and duration: long-lasting, and commonly suboccipital, associated with sustained contraction of skeletal muscles, usually as a part of the individual's reaction during life-stress."[7]

When tension headaches are combined with a vascular type of headache they are termed "combined headaches," which are essentially "combinations of vascular headache of the migraine type and muscle contraction headache," both prominently coexisting in an attack.[8]

Despite attempts to differentiate headaches of vascular etiology from headaches resulting from muscular tension, electromyographic (EMG) studies of muscle contraction have been noted during migraines or migraine variants. However, these EMG findings are inconsistent in tension headaches, creating a paradox.[9]

To the average clinician a tension headache is characterized by its frequency cycle and is a disorder without a vascular component, that is, without prodrome or scotoma. It is usually provoked by stress or emotional factors. There have been so many inconclusive terms applied to this diagnosis that it is considered by many to be a wastebasket diagnosis.[10]

There are numerous headaches that are not classically vascular, are not associated with identifiable organic structural disease, and occur in the presence of stress, anxiety, depression, anger, or even prolonged positional postural changes. They have been termed *tension myalgia* and allegedly constitute 12 percent of the 5000 patients a year seen at the Mayo Clinic Department of Physical Medicine.[11]

With tension headache occurring as often as it does, this diagnostic entity must be accepted as a factual occurrence even though not as an "illness." Pain usually alerts the person of an impending illness or injury, but the symptom of pain may also protect people from emotional or mental stress or trauma.

Pain has been called the third emotion, the other two being anxiety and depression.[12] Admittedly mild in most cases, tension headaches may become severe, persistent, disabling, and treatment-resistant. The mechanism of tension headaches is postulated to occur from the tender spots within the afflicted muscles and transmitted to the central nervous system through the $A = \alpha$ and C fibers of the trigeminal nerve and the upper three cervical roots and possibly via the sympathetic nervous system.[13] Once in the dorsal columns of the cord, these fibers ascend and ultimately reach the thalamus, with all its ramifications.

Throughout the ascension through the spinal cord and the midbrain and into the cortex, many factors modulate the nociceptive impulses; some of these are cultural, learned, and emotionally charged. All these factors that enhance or inhibit the intensity and interpretation of the ultimate pain are central in the cord and midbrain and are ultimately cortical. But they are initiated, modified, and maintained at the peripheral muscle level. These factors of pain modulation will be extensively discussed in Chapter 11.

Myofascial Pain Syndrome

Myofascial pain, fibrositis, or fibromyalgia all have headache as an associated symptom (see Chapter 7). This suggests that one or several muscle groups of the head or muscles attached to the head must be involved and that these muscles generate the nociceptor reactions (see Fig. 4–1).

Acute Tension Headache

Acute tension headache is conceived as a solitary episode of headache termed as "tension" by the patient. The headache is considered as being muscular in etiology and occurs following a sustained postural position, an acute emotional episode, or an otherwise stressful and emotionally fatiguing activity.

The symptoms are usually described as a sensation of tightness in the head, a "band around the head," usually predominantly in the occipital-frontal region.

These attacks are usually termed mild in that they do not significantly limit activities to a measurable degree. They respond to anti-inflammatory medication such as aspirin. Muscle relaxants are effective, and modalities such as massage, gentle traction, ice packs, or heat packs are beneficial.

Recurrent Tension Headache

The term *recurrent tension headache* is probably more appropriate than the term *chronic tension headache*, although they each imply the same situation. Treatment is usually that of addressing the acute episode, but the major emphasis should be on prevention of another attack. This involves identifying causative factors and elucidating the personality that allows these factors to produce an attack. If a personality factor or particular source of stress seem causative, counseling, biofeedback, aerobic exercises, yoga, meditation, self-hypnosis, and other stress management techniques have all proven effective. The need for such techniques depends on the severity, the resultant disability, the anxiety of a possible recurrence, the fear of these attacks progressing into another more disabling disease, and the patient's acceptance of the relationship between tension and stress and the headaches. Some of these programs are expensive and require time and patient compliance—factors that must be considered by the physician and the patient.

As most of these headaches are disturbing but not life-threatening, this fact must be carefully and thoroughly explained to the patient. Many physicians consider that alleviating fear is a major aspect of tension headache treatment.[14] Reassurance is mandatory and this begins with the proper use of a diagnostic label—one that the patient understands and accepts. Compliance is therefore more readily assured.[15]

The term *tension myalgia* has been considered valid in that tension can be explained as a physiological state, not a psychological state.[16] "All in your

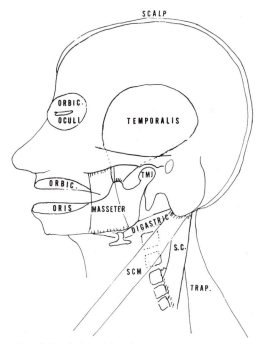

Figure 4–1. Muscles of the face and head.

The major muscles of the face and head that may be sites of myalgia (muscular pain). The list is inconclusive.

The temporalis muscle originates from the temporal fossa, passes under the arch, and attaches to the coronoid process of the mandible, which it elevates upon contraction. It is also involved in TMJ arthralgia. TMJ is the temporomandibular joint.

The masseter muscle originates from the zygomatic arch and attaches to the superior margin of the ramus of the mandible. Its action is to close the mouth.

The orbicularis muscles are muscles of facial expression: The oculi close the eyes and the oris the mouth. The digastric muscle originates from the mastoid notch to attach to the inferior border of the mandible. It depresses the mandible and elevates the hyoid bone.

Muscles that attach to the skull are splenius capitis (SC), which goes from the midline fascia of the cervical vertebrae to attach to the mastoid process; the sternocleidomastoid muscle (SCM), at this site of insertion upon the mastoid; and the upper trapezius muscles (Trap).

head" is not implied. Tension in a muscle is understood by a patient as being a contracted muscle that becomes fatigued and may ache from this sustained shortening. The value of modalities such as stretching exercises, heat, and ice become evident when the patient understands the physiology of a contracted muscle. Biofeedback indicates that the contraction of an "offending" muscle can be brought under voluntary conscious control of the patient. The patient becomes a "member of the treatment team" and actively involved in the treatment process.

Myalgia can also be explained to the patient in acceptable terms as a correctable "condition" of a muscle, not a disease. The ultimate use of tricyclic antidepressants (TCA) can also be explained as being used for their "chemical rebalancing" and not merely for treating depression. To avoid overmedication or dependency, an explanation of the indications and contraindications for NSAIDs is also needed. Preventive medications play a role. Tricyclic antidepressants have become a valid and effective approach even though overt depression may not be evident or accepted by the patient. Their pharmacological action has a serotonin action, which may be the basis for their effectiveness. TCAs also rebalance the sleep cycle which is so often impaired in these chronic daily headache patients.[17]

The recommended dosage of TCA medication is bedtime medication beginning in small doses and increasing as indicated to an effective, tolerated, and beneficial dose. The addition of a beta blocker (propranolol and nadolol) to TCA is also effective, as is NSAID medication. These drugs are addictive and require both careful monitoring and patient and family compliance.

Patients who experience recurrent periodic headaches are often difficult to manage. They have a tendency to misuse or overuse medication, have personal and family stresses, and are often noncompliant with the prescribed program. A comprehensive approach is required including all the above modalities outlined.

MUCOSAL MEMBRANE SITE OF HEAD AND NECK PAIN

Less frequently seen in general practice than head and face pain, mucosal pain must be recognized and addressed as it has more serious implications. This is also the head pain self-diagnosed by patients with inappropriate treatment. Many patients with headache attribute their symptoms to "sinus trouble," nasal congestion, etc., and self-medicate with no benefit and often significant addiction and side effects. The vast array of over-the-counter medications found in the average drugstore attests to this propensity.

Except for the dorsum of the anterior two-thirds of the tongue, the oral cavity and the anterior chamber of the nasal cavity, paranasal sinuses, and the nasopharyngeal regions are lined with stratified squamous epithelium and are supplied by salivary and mucous glands. These fibrous tissues are amply supplied by neurovascular innervation.

Their afferent pain fibers are transmitted through the ophthalmic, maxillary, and mandibular divisions of the trigeminal nerve, whose cell bodies are located in the gasserian ganglion. The peripheral nociceptors are immediately below the epithelium with some fiber endings located in deeper connective tissues and the vascular walls. The posterior tongue, which has no mucosa, has its pain fiber impulses transmitted via the glossopharyngeal trunk.

The peripheral nociceptor endings are affected by viral, bacterial, and fungal infections as well as autoimmune disease processes. Vesiculations, ulcerations, and gradual atrophy of these mucosal tissues can result. Obstructive salivary and mucosal gland conditions also occur, which result in oral, nasal, and facial pain.

Viral Vesicular Mucositis

There are three viruses that are primarily responsible for painful vesicular eruption in the mucosal tissues. These are herpes simplex, varicella-zoster virus, and Coxsackievirus. When these viruses are involved they create constitutional symptoms as well as local manifestations, including fever, lymphadenopathy, generalized malaise, and mucosal pain and hypersensitivity. The latter is both diagnostic and the most incapacitating. Many of these infections cause an eruption of vesicals which cast suspicion as to their etiology.

Most viral infections run their natural course in 10 to 14 days, but they have the tendency to recur. Some, besides being mucosal in the nares and oral cavities, are also in the genital mucosa. Nearly 98 percent of the population over 21 years harbor antibodies of HSV type 1 and 15 to 20 percent of adults have a history of recurrent herpes labialis.[18]

Viral Pharyngitis

This pharyngitis considered to be viral in etiology is the common cold in which there are general systemic disabling symptoms and an erythematous pharynx, mucopurulent rhinorrhea, a low grade fever, and even lymphadenopathy.

Bacterial Mucosal Infections

Bacterial mucosal infections are infrequent except for the occasional odontogenic or periodontal infections. In bacterial mucosal infections it is probably a secondary infection in conjunction with viral infection such as in stomatitis, laryngitis, pharyngitis, rhinitis, and sinusitis.

The systemic symptoms of infection and inflammation accompanied by mucosal lesions (vesicle, ulceration, erythema, and local pain and tenderness) indicate the disease process causing the facial and head pain syndrome, and their treatment is supportive of antibiotic and antiviral medication. Failure to abort or eradicate the offending infectious agent may lead to chronic infection that becomes resistant to the use of further antibiotics. Consultation by an otolaryngologist may be needed as well as specific culture testing, but the diagnosis of these conditions being the source of face and head pain initiates the diagnostic process.

Fungal Infections of Mucosal Tissues

The most common mycotic infection of the upper respiratory tract is candidiasis (*Candida albicans*), but this fungus infection rarely affects people who are otherwise healthy. It usually occurs in a person who is otherwise debilitated with another type of infection or illness. Even when the infection is corrected by antibiotics the fungus may proliferate. The infection results in papules containing a milky fluid that becomes diagnostic on smears sent to the laboratory.

Treatment of a mucosal fungus is topical nystatin or oral troches of chlortrimizole. Ketoconazole orally (200 mgm/d) has proven effective. Fungus infections frequently occur from chronic use of ill-fitting dentures, a circumstance which can be corrected with proper dental orthosis.

Allergic Mucositis

There are numerous allergens that affect the mucosa such as pollens, foodstuffs, mouthwashes, etc. This allergic reaction causes erythema and edema of the mucous membranes with pain, obstructive respiratory symptoms, and some secretions. This mucosal reaction responds to antihistamines, nasal decongestants, and antibiotics to prevent secondary infection.

Erythema Multiformis

Although this disease is primarily a dermatological condition, it does involve the mucous membranes of the nose and mouth. When erythema multiforme results from sensitivity to a drug it may be sufficiently serious to not only eliminate the offending drug (allergen) but to institute steroid therapy: prednisone 40 to 60 mgm/d for 7 to 10 days.

There is a voluminous literature regarding the diagnosis and treatment of viral, bacterial, fungus, and allergic mucosal lesions that the reader may refer to but that will not be enumerated in this text.[18]

OTALGIA

Pain in the head region may be caused by ear pathology emanating from the ear proper or regions about the ear.

The ear is neurologically supplied by the trigeminal, facial, glossopharyngeal, and vagus nerves. Its sensory distribution is from the C-2 to C-3 branches of the cervical plexus (see Chapter 1). In summary , the anterior aspect of the external ear receives its innervation from the auriculotemporal nerve, a branch of the mandibular division of the trigeminal nerve. The posterior surface of the external ear is supplied by the greater occipital nerve (C-3). The floor of the auditory canal receives innervation from the auricular branch of the vagus nerve. This innervation explains why reflex coughing occurs often during an examination of the inner ear. The posterior aspect of the ear canal receives supply from the facial nerve.

The tympanic membrane is innervated by branches of the glossopharyngeal nerve as well as being amply supplied by sympathetic nerves. With such an intense innervation it is apparent why ear pathology causes pain in that region of the head and face.

Infections of the Ear Canal

Acute otitis externa is either bacterial or fungal and may result from excessive moisture, as in swimmer's ear or from minor trauma. Symptoms vary from mild ache to excruciating pain with possible loss of hearing. Examination reveals redness and edema of the external canal, possible discharge, and pain on passive movement of the external ear.

Treatment includes topical antibiotics after cleaning and suctioning of the debris and discharge. If there is extreme swelling with partial occlusion of the canal, a wick soaked with antibiotic can be inserted into the canal and allowed to remain several days. Systemic antibiotics are rarely indicated unless there is also systemic symptomatology and adenopathy.

Fungal infections of the canal cause a sensation of fullness and itching, but not necessarily pain. Hearing may be impaired if the canal becomes mechanically blocked by debris.

The most common fungi are *Aspergillis niger* or *Candida albicans*, causing a creamy white discharge. Treatment consists of antifungal ear drops either with or without desiccating drops of boric acid and alcohol.

If the infestation is pseudomonas it can be severe and lead to complications. Indicators include failure to respond to the usual treatment and granulomatous tissue within the canal at the bony cartilaginous junction. It is the proximity to the bone that makes this infection ominous as it presents the possibility of osteomyelitis. Treatment is administration of oral anti-pseudomona antibiotics and even intravenous antibiotics and antifungicides.

Middle Ear Infections

Acute inner ear infections are termed otitis media and present as an acute onset of ear pain, fever, a feeling of a sense of fullness in the ear, and a loss of hearing. The physical examination reveals a red and possibly bulging tympanic membrane. If the infection has existed for a period of time the membrane may have ruptured and a bloody purulent discharge may be present. When rupture has occurred, the pain decreases or subsides.

Treatment is identification of the offending organism and use of antibiotics after culture and sensitivity studies. Failure to abort the early infection may result in mastoiditis, meningitis, and other septic effects such as abscesses.

Chronic otitis is usually painless and presents primarily as chronic drainage, loss of hearing, and even bony erosion of the canal.

Orofacial pain may result from inner and outer ear infection, but its proximity to the temporomandibular joint makes the relationship apparent as to the pain emanating from the TMJ and/or the ear. Proximity of the teeth to the ear also makes dental pathology suspect in assuming the pain to be from auricular pathology. The parotid gland is also in close proximity, and it or thyroiditis may relate to ear pain.[19]

PARANASAL SINUS HEADACHE AND FACIAL PAIN

Infection, inflammation, and obstruction of the paranasal sinuses are a cause of head and facial pain. Many patients erroneously attribute their headaches to "sinus," but when there is a relationship the pain is specifically located in the region of the involved sinus. Multiple involved sinus infections cause a diffuse headache not necessarily related to the involved sinuses. The obstruction of infected sinuses undoubtedly causes local pain as well as generalized head and face pain.

The symptoms attributed to sinus disease are usually characterized as dull, nonpulsating pain exaggerated by head movements, coughing, and sneezing. They may be vague and overlap the entire spectrum of generalized headache. Chronic frontal sinusitis is usually more painful than acute sinusitis.

SINUS HEADACHE

Patients suffering from sinus headache usually have had a history of preceding upper respiratory infection. There is pain and tenderness in the distribution of the trigeminal nerve and examination reveals engorgement of the nasal turbinates, erythema with possible discharge. If the sinus involved is the frontal sinus there may be severe pain and tenderness from direct pressure over the frontal sinus area. Routine x-rays may reveal haziness of the sinuses, but MRI and CT scan appear more reliable as a diagnostic procedure.

The reason that sinus disease is difficult to document as the primary cause of head pain is that any referred pain of the maxillary and ophthalmic divisions of the trigeminal nerve mimic the pain of sinus disease. Specific noxious stimulus of the nasal cavity creates a referred headache pain.[20] Noxious stimulus to the inferior turbinate refers pain to the upper teeth, the zygoma, and the eye. Noxious stimulus to the middle turbinate refers pain to the temple area, the zygoma, the inner canthus of the eye, and the forehead. There is such an overlap of neuronal connection in the cord and central nervous system that confusion of the specific mechanism of facial pain resulting from sinus disease results.[21]

OCULAR PAIN

Ocular pain, pain about or within the eye orbit, is the most common site of head and face pain. Pain associated with primary eye disease has been called *primary ophthalmic headache*.[22] Pain within the eye may be associated by pain around the eye socket (periorbital) and with concurrent headache and even scalp pain and contractures. This type of headache should be recognized as a primary ocular pathology in order to avoid permanent visual impairment.

Pain about the eye (periocular) with no apparent intrinsic eye disease presents the major problem here. The eye is a well-established site for referred pain from elsewhere in the face and head. It behooves the physician to explore the specific eye condition before blandly treating the condition as generalized face and head pain "incidentally affecting the eye region." The eye may present conjunctival congestion and lacrimation and yet be unassociated with pathology elsewhere, such as sinusitis, etc. Discrimination is mandated when the eye or the eye region is involved in a patient claiming subjective headache or face pain.

A careful history, as has been discussed, should narrow the potential sites of the professed head and face pain and the examination must include a thorough, comprehensive eye examination.

Primary Ocular Pathology Causing Pain

Local eye disease must follow a schematic protocol of examining the eye beginning anteriorly and progressing within the depth of the eye: lids, conjunctiva, cornea, sclera, iris, ciliary body, retina, optic nerve, and structures within the orbit. Any of these structures may be the site of pain and disability.

Lids. The lids can be simply examined by direct vision and upward (downward) reflection. Major sources of lid pain are acute infection of the lacrimal gland (styes) or chronic inflammation of these glands (halazion). Swelling is noted with inflammation, crusting, and associated conjunctival inflammation. These usually present symptoms of burning or stinging, mostly upon awakening; often the eyelids are matted together. Painful involuntary eye closure may occur (blepharospasm).

Treatment is local cleansing with a warm saline solution or baby shampoo. Local infiltration (drops or swabs) of topical antibiotic solution or even mild steroid ocular solutions afford relief and recovery.

Conjunctiva. Inflammation and infection of the conjunctiva cause pain, tearing, itching, burning, and even blepharitis. Because the conjunctiva is minimally innervated, it usually presents more with objective signs than with subjective complaints of pain. The presence of conjunctival inflammation with significant pain should alert the examiner to look for other more ominous eye problems.

Cornea. The cornea is the most densely innervated tissue of the body and hence is also exquisitely sensitive. Any irritation causes severe local pain, lacrimation, photophobia, blepharospasm, and radiation of pain into the forehead and periorbital area.

If trauma with possible ulceration is suspected a drop of fluorescein will highlight the ulceration to direct ophthalmoscopic examination. A drop of topical anesthetic (Tetracaine or Ophthaine) will also decrease the pain immediately as well as be diagnostic in that the pain perceived by the patient emanates from the cornea.

Corneal abrasions or ulcerations are usually self-limited and, after the removal of a foreign body, heal within a few days. Antibiotic and anesthetic drops with an eye patch relieve the pain and permit healing, usually within days.

In the elderly or debilitated patient the presence of dry eyes can be a source of pain or significant discomfort. When combined with a dry mouth the possibility of Sjögen's syndrome, a rheumatological disease variant, must be entertained. Because dry eyes also enhance the possibility of ulceration as well as being a source of discomfort eye drops several times daily are indicated.

Uvea. The uvea is the middle coat of the eye—the iris, anterior chamber contents, ciliary body, and posterior choroid. Only the ciliary body is amply innervated.[23]

Uveitis is either infectious or granulomatous. Symptoms of uveitis are pain, significant photophobia, diminution of vision with "presence of particles floating in the anterior chamber." The eye is tender to the touch, and there is a possible irregularity of pupillary response to light. Photophobia is determined by the patient's reaction to a light during the examination. Treatment requires placing the internal eye at rest by installation of cycloplegic dilators.

Lens. In the presence of glaucoma, the pupil is fixed in midpoint, there may be a degree of visual loss, a mild headache may occur, and increased occular pressure may gradually cause optic atrophy.[24] To check for glaucoma, test the ocular pressure. If there is pain in a patient with chronic glaucoma, other inflammatory conditions must be sought.

Retina. Pain occurring from exposure to light (photophobia) from retinitis is thought to occur from ciliary body contraction, but this concept is refuted by failure to relieve the pain by installation of cycloplegic drops. If there is severe photophobia but no clearly identifiable pathology, the patient should consult an ophthalmologist.

Optic Nerve. The pain that results from optic neuritis is painful loss of vision and impaired acuity, color perception, and full visual field.[25] The subjective loss of vision with diminution or loss of peripheral visual fields may indicate a retrobulbar neuritis, the onset of multiple sclerosis, or other forms of demyelinating diseases and requires evaluation by a neuro-ophthalmologist or neurologist. Steroids have proven disappointing and may lull the practitioner into failing to do adequate studies to determine the exact cause of optic neuritis.[26]

Eye Orbit. The orbit is a closed container adjacent to many sinuses and therefore may present secondary symptoms and findings that belong elsewhere. The presence of clinical signs such as lid swelling, erythema, warmth, and pain may indicate adjacent sinus inflammation. CT scan may reveal the precise site and degree of sinusitis so that appropriate antibiotics may be prescribed. The value of MRI in sinusitis remains as yet imprecise.

In evaluating ocular disease as the cause of headache it must be stated that there are painful ocular diseases that present minimal or no objective signs upon examination and suggest further studies.

Eye Strain as a Cause of Headache

Headache from eyestrain enjoys a popularity that may be unjustified yet causes numerous visits to optometrists and ophthalmologists.[27] "Eyestrain" occurs from frontal muscle tension and possibly even blurred vision. Muscle imbalance may cause discomfort but correction of the imbalance may also fail to eliminate the headache. Treatment is obviously the treatment of the headache, not the visual aspect.

There are undoubtedly other numerous ocular conditions that relate to concurrent headaches but cannot be enumerated in this text. Suffice to say that if ocular symptoms fail to respond to treatment or continue to concern the practitioner or the patient, the patient should consult an ophthalmologist.

REFERENCES

1. Harris, L and Associates: The Nuprin Pain Report, A National Study Conducted for Nuprin. No. 851017. New York, September 1985, pp 1–19.
2. Kanner, AD, Coyne, JC, Schaefer, C, and Lazarus, RS: Comparison of two modes of stress measurement: Daily hassles and uplifts versus major life events. J Behav Med 4(1): 1–39, 1981.
3. Dalessio, DJ: Physician health study. JAMA (in press) 1991.
4. Tfelt-Hansen, P and Olesen, J.: Effervescent metoclopramide and aspirin vs. effervescent aspirin or placebo for migraine attacks: A double-blind study. Cephalalgia 4:107–111, 1984.
5. Ward, N, Whitney, C, Avery, D, and Dunner, D: The analgesic effects of caffeine in headache. Pain 44:151–155, 1991.
6. Bond, MR: Personality and pain. In Bond, MR: Pain: Its Nature, Analysis and Treatment, ed 2. Churchill Livingstone, London, 1984, pp 45–50.
7. Ad Hoc Committee on Classification of Headache. Arch Neurol 6:173–176, 1963.
8. Dalession, DJ: Wolff's Headache. Oxford University Press, New York, 1980.
9. Pikoff, H: Is the muscular model of headache still viable? A review of conflicting data. Headache 24:186–198, 1984.
10. Saper, JR: Changing perspective on chronic headache. Clin J Pain 2:19–28, 1986.
11. Stonnington, HH: Tension myalgia. Mayo Clin Proc 52:750–751, 1977.
12. Swanson, DW: Chronic pain as a third pathologic emotion. Am J Psych 141:210–214, 1984.
13. Olesen, J and Langemark, M: Mechanisms of tension headache: A speculative hypothesis. In Olesen, J and Edvinsson, L (eds): Basic Mechanisms of Headache, Vol 2. Elsevier, Amsterdam, 1988, pp 457–461.
14. Kori, SH, Miller, RP, and Todd, DD: Kinisophobia: A new view of chronic pain behavior. Pain Management Jan–Feb:35–43, 1990.
15. Turk, DC and Rudy, TE: Neglected topics in the treatment of chronic pain patients—relapse, noncompliance and adherence enhancement. Pain 44:5–28, 1991.
16. Thompson, JM: Subspecialty clinics: Physical medicine and rehabilitation: Tension myalgia as a diagnosis at the Mayo Clinic and its relationship to fibrositis, fibromyalgia and myofascial pain syndrome. Mayo Clin Proc 65:1237–1248, 1990.
17. Mathew, NT, Glaze, D, and Frost, J: Sleep apnea and other sleep abnormalities in primary headache disorders. In Rose, C (ed): Migraine Procedures. Fifth International Migraine Symposium, London (1989), pp 48–49 (Krager), Basel (1985).
18. Eversole, LR: Mucosal pain disorders of the head and neck. In Jacobson, AL and Donion, WC (eds): Headache and Facial Pain. Raven Press, New York, 1990, pp 53–80.
19. Wazen, J and Abramson, M: In English, G (ed): Otolaryngology. JB Lippincott, Philadelphia, 1989.
20. Greenfield, H: Presented at the meeting of the American Academy of Otolaryngology, San Antonio, Texas, September 1986. Quoted in Rosenblum, BM and Friedman, WH: Paranasal sinus etiologies of headache and facial pain, Chap 10. In Jacobson, AL and Donion, WC (eds): Headache and Facial Pain. Raven Press, New York, pp 235–244, 1990.
21. Ibid: Etiologies of headache and facial pain, Chap 10. In Jacobson, AL and Donion, WC (eds): Headache and Facial Pain. Raven Press, New York, 1990 pp 243.
22. Troost, T: In Lessell, S and Delenes, JT (eds): Current Neuroophthalmology, Vol 1. Year Book Medical Publishers, Chicago, 1988, pp 269–287.
23. Friedman, AH, Luntz, M, and Henley, WL: Diagnosis and Management of Uveitis. Williams & Wilkins, Baltimore, 1985, p 115.
24. Zuazo, A, Ibanez, J, and Belmote, C: Exp Eye Res 43:759–769, 1986.
25. Burde, RM, Savino, PJ, and Trobe, JD: Clinical Decisions in Neuroophthalmology. CV Mosby, St Louis, 1985, pp 35–40.
26. Cox, TA and Woolson, RF: Arch Ophthamol 99:338, 1981.
27. Cameron, ME: Med J Austral 1:292–294, 1976.

CHAPTER 5

Chronic Facial Pains: Neuralgias

The patient with chronic facial pain presents a quandary to the practitioner as to management. The symptoms of facial pain must be addressed by a meticulous search for the correct diagnosis before initiating cursory symptomatic treatment. There are a few major facial pains, but the more frequent "atypical" face pains that confront the clinician may portend an ominous etiology.

The classification of chronic facial pains is listed in Table 5–1. It is nonconclusive but gives a reasonable differential diagnosis for the clinician. We will discuss some of the more common neuralgias.

TRIGEMINAL NEURALGIA

This is a severe acute-onset facial pain that usually strikes after the age of 30 unless it is a sequela of multiple sclerosis, in which case it can occur at any age. The areas of intense pain are in the distribution of the trigeminal nerve (see Fig. 1–2) and are usually about the nares. These indicated sites are accompanied by the presence of trigger zones: areas of skin of exquisite sensitivity to touch. These areas, per se sensitive, are also the sites that initiate an attack when touched or irritated in any manner.

The patient presenting with this potential diagnosis characterizes the pain by assiduously avoiding any touch of the face when washing, shaving, biting, chewing, or even smiling. In many facial painful conditions the opposite is usually observed, in that the patient frequently massages, rubs, or applies heat or ice to the face to receive benefit. Not allowing any touch or exposure is actually diagnostic of probable trigeminal neuralgia.

**Table 5–1. CLASSIFICATION OF CHRONIC
FACIAL PAINS**

  I. Muscular
        Myositis
        Fibromyalgia
        Neoplastic
 II. Neuritic
        Paroxysmal
          Trigeminal neuralgia
          Glossopharyngeal neuralgia
        Chronic
          Posttraumatic
          Postherpetic
          Toxic
        Multiple sclerosis
III. Rheumatic
        Secondary to collagen disease
        Temporomandibular
        Infectious
        Neoplastic
 IV. Vascular
        Paroxysmal recurrent
          Migraine
          Migraine variant
          Cluster headache
          Cluster variant
        Toxic metabolic
        Hypertensive
        Arterial
          Atherosclerosis
          Embolic
          Aneurysmal
          Arteriovenous malformation
          Transient ischemic attack (TIA)
        Thrombophlebitis
        Arteritis
          Giant cell
          Granulomatous/infectious
          Immune complex
  V. Psychogenic
        Conversion hysteria
        Depression equivalent
        Atypical face pain
 VI. Dental, Oral, Mucosal, Ocular, Otalgic

An attack is usually described as "jabbing or stabbing" in nature and lasts 20 to 30 seconds. This attack is typically followed by a brief period (several seconds) of relief, only to be followed by another stabbing attack. Attacks of longer duration are rarely if ever typically present.[1,2]

The pathophysiology of trigeminal neuralgia presumes that there is a period of build up of nerve sensitivity probably located in the brain stem (pons) circuits (see Fig. 1–2). These circuits include the spinal nucleus of the Vth cranial nerve. There is also probably a peripheral mechanism in that the trigeminal nerve is also sensitized. The causes or the precise manner of these sensitizations centrally and peripherally remain conjectural and may be chemical nociceptors occurring from varied causes and in a susceptible host.

The frequent presence of trigeminal neuralgia in multiple sclerosis (MS) (1 to 2 percent of patients) also fails to clarify or confirm the causative agent because in this neurological demyelinating disease the involved nerve becomes hypersensitive in an area that is frequently hypoalgesic (numb or anesthetized).[3] The area that becomes the site of a jabbing sensation objectively exhibits hyperesthesia, hyperalgesia, and loss of temperature sensation. In MS the corneal reflex may be absent if the first division of the trigeminal nerve is involved.

As a rule the presence of trigeminal neuralgia usually does not occur in the first episode of MS but is noted in later and more developed neurological impairment of the disease. In pathological studies of MS patients suffering from trigeminal neuralgia regions of demyelination have been found in the gasserian nucleus, the facial nerve, and the Vth cranial nerve as it enters the brain stem. Similar studies in non-MS patients are not found in the literature. Thus demyelination is not considered pertinent, nor is its presence helpful in determining the etiology of pain.

Medication

The medical treatment of a confirmed trigeminal neuralgia is to interrupt the buildup of the afferent impulses which are considered to ultimately trigger the abrupt acute attack. In susceptible patients the region of the trigeminal nerve becomes sensitive to touch or air and indicates a pending attack.

Generally, the treatment of a trigeminal neuralgia is begun with the administration of carbamazepine (Tegretol oral tabs) 100 to 200 mgm b.i.d. or t.i.d. If the acute attack is terminated and this drug dosage is tolerated by the patient, the drug is continued for several weeks or months. A maintenance dose of 200 mgm daily usually suffices, but this must be monitored for the specific patient and the response as well as tolerance of the drug.

Besides clinical monitoring to evaluate effectiveness and tolerance, the serum level of the administered drug can be determined with the attempt being to maintain a level of carbamazepine at 6 to 12 μg/mL.

If given early carbamazepine (Tegretol), essentially an anticonvulsant, can abrupt the summation leading to an attack.[4,5] If this drug does not abort the attack within 24 to 48 hours the diagnosis is considered to be questionable. It must be remembered that the diagnosis is made primarily from the history and reproduction of exquisite sensitivity to the dermatomal area of the trigeminal nerve, and thus a subjective response to medication that is considered specific is diagnostic as well as therapeutic.

Use of carbamazepine may prophylactically control further attacks, and after treatment of acute attacks further follow-up with medication may no longer be necessary. If there is recurrence that responds poorly to this medication, other drugs can be tried. Carbamazepine may cause unpleasant side effects, such as unacceptable sedation, and thus be rejected by the patient. This also may imply the need for other medications. These other drugs can be added to carbamazepine when the therapeutic dose and acquired blood level fails to deter attacks. Other drugs include the following:

Baclofen (Lioresal) 10 mgm daily is initially employed and gradually increased to 60 to 80 mg daily at 3- to 5-day intervals in divided doses. These drugs, which were initially considered effective in decreasing the spasticity of upper motor neurone disease such as stroke, MS, spinal cord injury, etc., are also effective in decreasing painful neuralgias.

Diphenylhydantoin (Dilantin) 200 to 400 mgm daily or *chlorphenesin* (Maolate) 800 to 2400 mgm daily may be added to, or used in place, of carbamazepine. If all three are needed and cause undesirable side effects, such as sedation, weakness, and hemopoiesis, surgical intervention can be suggested. The use of two drugs (e.g., chlorphenesin and diphenylhydantoin) is certainly to be tried before deciding that drug medication will not be effective.

The pharmacological mechanisms of all these drugs are similar. They reduce the post-tetanic potentiation of transmission across synapses within the cord and at the sympathetic ganglia synopsis. (Post-tetanic potentiation is the enhancement of transmission across a synapse which follows rapid, repetitive presynaptic stimulation.[6]) Studies have also shown this depression at the spinal cord nucleus.[4] It is apparently what causes the irritable neurone effect of the disease to be effectively diminished and thus prevent buildup resulting in an attack.

Surgical Treatment

As stated above, the drugs used to treat or prevent trigeminal attacks can cause drowsiness, dizziness, and generalized weakness. The depression of central nervous system activity may cause speech slurring, diplopia, ataxia, and even nystagmus. Any of these are an indication for discontinuing the medication. Nausea and vomiting may also occur and, if uncontrollable, may also indicate need for discontinuing the drug.

When all attempts of medical treatment of trigeminal neuralgia fail, a surgical procedure may need to be considered. Excision of a wide section of the nerve is now rarely performed, but there are other procedures.

The trigeminal nerve can be interrupted by being injected with a glycerol solution.[7] Or it can be ablated with a radio frequency electrode.[8,9] This is a relatively simple and safe procedure, done with a light anesthesia, and can be performed with the patient awake. Recovery is rapid and hospitalization is usually needed only with overnight observation. Complications include the persistence of uncomfortable dysesthesias, corneal anesthesia, jaw musculature weakness, and a possible recurrence (25 percent of operated patients).[8] Most of these surgical residuals can be tolerated by the patient who has suffered intractable neuralgia, but they must be carefully discussed with the patient before the procedure is undertaken so there is no postoperative concern and in today's society, no litigation.

GLOSSOPHARYNGEAL NEURALGIA

Clinically similar in most ways to trigeminal neuralgia, an attack of glossopharyngeal neuralgia is an abrupt, acute, severe attack of pain in the region of the tonsil and ear.[10] Like trigeminal neuralgia it can be triggered by swallowing, contact of food with the tonsillar area, or even yawning. The nasopharynx area in which the pain is perceived is not sensitive to touch between attacks nor hyperalgesic or hyperesthetic to touch or pinprick. As with other similar neuralgias, the diagnosis is made by history and by response to medication.

Treatment

Carbamazepine (Tegretol) orally is usually effective. The same doses are indicated as for trigeminal neuralgia, and the initial treatment should be followed by a maintenance dose for several weeks. As in the trigeminal neuralgia, if the carbamazepine is ineffective or inadequate diphenylhydantoin or baclofen can be added before nerve-interruptive procedures are considered.

The simplest and often effective treatment to abort or relieve an attack of glossopharyngeal neuralgia after failure of the above drugs is the cocainization of the involved side of the throat. This can be applied by coating the throat region with a large cotton swab containing a cocaine solution.

Upon failure of all more conservative procedures and in the presence of recurrent severe attacks, a surgical interruption is indicated. This is an invasive intracranial procedure of which the surgical details will not be fully discussed in this text. It involves a craniotomy to locate and identify the nerve as it passes along the floor of the posterior fossa. The nerve ultimately emerges through the jugular foramen.

POSTHERPETIC NEURITIC NEURALGIA

One of the more severe but not necessarily the most frequent, neuralgias resulting from the herpetic viral invasion is of significant disability and it deserves emphasis.

There have been many reports of the pathology of the postherpetic nerve lesion, but it still remains to be fully elucidated.[11,12] The current concept is the microscopic findings of fibrosis and cell loss in the dorsal root ganglion.[13] The sensory nerve fibers especially show demyelination, and there is concommittent demyelination in the dorsal horn of the spinal cord at those segments. Some fibrosis and loss of nerve fibers have also been reported within the peripheral nerve of the involved segment.

Herpetic lesions without pain have also revealed these pathological changes, implying that there must be other forms of inflammation in patients with herpetic pain.[14] This explains the benefit from use of steroids in the acute phase.

GIANT CELL ARTERITIS

Temporal arteritis is only one of the numerous types of necrotizing arteritis conditions. These painful conditions are characterized by segmental inflammation of medium- and small-sized blood vessels. The pathology is an infiltration of polymorphonuclear leukocytes and eosinophils within the walls of the involved arteries, resulting in thrombosis and segmental fibrinoid necrosis.[15]

In giant cell arteritis the inflammation is more chronic, with granulomatous changes which, when they heal by fibrosis within the wall and adventia, cause a proliferation that may obstruct the vessel or lead to an obstructive aneurysmal dilatation.

This granulomatous arteritis may be generalized or focal. The initial systemic manifestations are fever, anorexia, weight loss, headache, fatigue, and myalgia. In cranial arteritis there is head pain localized over the temporal artery or widespread over the cranium, face, and jaws.[16] Painful tender nodules may be found in the scalp. The tender temporal artery may be devoid of pulsations.

Most patients are usually over 50 years of age and most commonly over

60. This condition occurs two to four times more frequently in women than in men. Pain is often not severe and, when present, is persistent not episodic.[17] The pain is described as steady aching rather than throbbing or pulsating. Often there is tenderness of the scalp and soreness even from the pressure of the pillow at bedtime. Because of its proximity to the temporomandibular joint, chewing may aggravate the pain.

This condition may be accompanied by ocular motor palsy with blindness from an optic neuropathy, occurring rapidly and usually irreversibly.[18] Loss of vision is the most feared sequela of this condition, especially in patients not diagnosed and appropriately treated. Vision can be lost in the other eye within a week of the initial affliction. Gradual blindness rather than abrupt visual loss is rare.

Associated symptoms should always be sought such as scalp tenderness, low grade fever, myalgia, painful facial swelling, ulcerations in the mouth, and anorexia.

The sedimentation rate (ESR) is characteristically elevated with leukocytosis, elevated α-2-globulin, and anemia. A biopsy is diagnostic.

Treatment is the early administration of high doses of oral steroids the minute the diagnosis is suspected. Failure to respond to this steroid administration argues against the diagnosis. Decreasing the high steroid dose too soon and too rapidly is contraindicated, as a remission may take years even with gradually tapering doses. The ESR determines the rate of remission.

REFERENCES

1. Fromm, GH: Trigeminal neuralgia-related disorders. Neurol Clin 7:305, 1989.
2. Fromm, GH, Terrance, CF, and Maroon, JC: Trigeminal neuralgia. Concepts regarding etiology and pathogenesis. Arch Neurol 41:1204, 1984.
3. Harris, W: Rare forms of paroxysmal trigeminal neuralgia and the relation to disseminated sclerosis. Br Med J 1:831, 1950.
4. Fromm, GH: Pharmacological consideration of anticonvulsants. Headache 9:35, 1969.
5. Fromm, GH: The pharmacology of trigeminal neuralgia. Clin Neuropharmacol 12:185, 1989.
6. Campbell, HJ: Correlative Physiology of the Nervous System. Academic Press, New York, 1965, pp 9–16.
7. Hakanson, S: Trigeminal neuralgia treated by injection of glycerol into the trigeminal cistern. Neurosurg 9:638, 1981.
8. Sweet, WH and Wepsic, JG: Controlled thermocoagulation of trigeminal ganglion and rootlets for differential destruction of pain fibers: I. Trigeminal neuralgia. J Neurosurg 40:143, 1974.
9. Tew, JM and Keller, JT: The treatment of trigeminal neuralgia by percutaneous radiofrequency technique. Clin Neurosurg 24:557, 1977.
10. Chawla, JC and Falconer, MA: Glossopharyngeal and vagal neuralgia. Br Med J 2:527, 1967.
11. Denny-Brown, D, Adams, RD, and Fitzgerald, PF: Pathologic features of herpes zoster: A note on geniculate herpes. Arch Neurol Psychiat 57:216, 1944.

12. Head, H and Campbell, AW: The pathology of herpes zoster and its bearing on sensory localization. Brain 23:353–523, 1900.
13. Zach, SI, Langfitt, TW, and Elliott, FA: Herpetic neuritis: A light and electron microscopic study. Neurology 14:744–750, 1964.
14. Watson, CPN, Morshead, C, Vander Kooy, D, and Evans, RJ: Post-herpetic neuralgia: Further post-mortem studies of cases with and without pain. Pain 44:105–117, 1991.
15. Arthritis Foundation: Primer on the rheumatic diseases, ed 7. JAMA 224(5):60–64, 1973.
16. Fauchaid, P, Rygvold, O, and Oystese, B: Temporal arteritis and polymyalgia rheumatica: Clinical and biopsy findings. Ann Intern Med 77:845–852, 1972.
17. Porta-Sales, J and Ferrer-Ruscalleda, F: Temporal ateritis. Present concepts. Cardivasc Rev Rep 6:310–321, 1985.
18. Jacobson, DM and Slamovits, TL: Erythrocyte sedimentation rate and its relationship to hematocrit in giant cell arteritis. Arch Ophthalmol 105:965–967, 1987.

CHAPTER 6

Head and Neck Pain from the Cervical Spine

The cervical spine has long been considered a major contributor to headache. Headache has been attributed to cervical degenerative disease, cervical tension, postural tension headaches, posttraumatic subluxations, osteophytes, etc. The term *cervicogenic headache* has received much medical consideration, yet the exact neurophysiological mechanism of cervicogenic headache remains totally unclear.[1] Many neurologists and rheumatologists deny the probability that headache can originate from the cervical spine.

Pain referred to the occipital region originating from the craniocervical region has been defined by the Ad Hoc Committee on Classification of Headache as "headache due to the spread of pain by noxious stimulation of other structures of the cranium and neck (periosteum, joint, ligament, muscle or cervical root)."[2] To make this diagnosis (craniocervical etiology), therefore, is justified only if the original nociceptive region as the cause of the headache can be ascertained to be the cervical spine and one of its tissues.[3]

The assertion of headache emanating from the cervical spine can only be substantiated if that specific headache can be reproduced by a specific cervical maneuver[4] or if it responds beneficially to treatment aimed exclusively at the cervical spine.[5] It does not suffice that the diagnosis of cervicogenic headache be made from the presence of radiological changes in the cervical spine. These changes are so frequent that their relationship to headache cannot be assumed. It also must be recognized that most radiological changes in the cervical spine are found in the lower cervical spine[6] and in most people past the age of 35 or 40, whereas headaches emanating from the cervical spine are mostly related to the upper cervical segments: the craniocervical spine.[5]

77

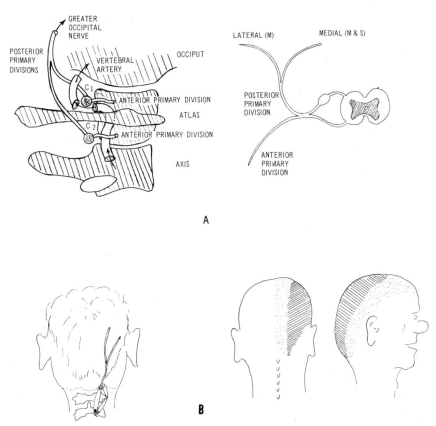

Figure 6–1. Occipital-atlanto-axis cervical region.

(A) The course of the C-1 and C-2 nerve roots that emerge to form the greater superior occipital nerve are depicted. The relationship to the vertebral artery is shown. (B) The dermatomal area of the nerve roots.

Headaches attributable to the cervical spine are usually in the region of the greater occipital cervical nerve unilateral or bilateral as it emerges from the cranial notch in the occipital region between the insertion of the trapezius and the sternocleidomastoid muscles (Figs. 6–1, 6–2). Pain in the occipital region is usually provoked by specific movements of the cervical spine and postural positions of the neck and head; it is associated with points of pressure tenderness that will reproduce the head pain.

Postinjury headaches are frequently attributed to cervical spine trauma in spite of as yet unconfirmed mechanism. This headache was termed "migraine cervicale" and was attributed to compression injury of the vertebral artery similar to the previously reported Barré syndrome.[7,8] The compression was attributed to vertebral subluxation of the upper cervical segment where the sympathetic fibers surrounding the vertebral artery are compressed in the

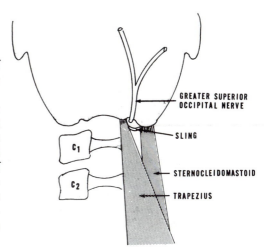

Figure 6–2. Occipital site of cranial emergence of the greater superior occipital nerve.

The greater superior occipital nerve, primarily C-2 nerve root emergence in a groove medial to the mastoid process between the sites of attachment of the sternocleidomastoid and the trapezius muscles. A fascial sling completes the opening through which the nerve emerges.

upper cervical region (see Fig. 6–1). This postulation attributes the headache to autonomic nervous origin.

A similar occipital headache accompanied by other autonomic symptoms also attributed occipital headache of cervical origin to autonomic nervous system imbalance.[9] This headache was relieved by local anesthetic blocking of the C-2 nerve root. This relationship, more recently discussed by Bogduk, will be discussed subsequently.[10]

TISSUE SITES OF CRANIOCERVICAL HEADACHE

The functional anatomy of the cervical spine must be reviewed and the relationship of the upper cervical nerve roots ascertained to postulate a resultant headache occurring.

Movement of the head upon the cervical spine occurs at the craniocervical junction: the occiput upon the atlas (Fig. 6–3). The atlas comprises two lateral bodies that articulate upon the occipital condyles (Fig. 6–4). Motion of this articulation is essentially 25 to 30° of flexion-extension. Little or no significant lateral or rotatory motion occurs between the occiput and the atlas.

The atlas articulates upon the axis (Fig. 6–5) and permits rotation about the odontoid process of approximately 45° in either direction (Fig. 6–6).

The cervical vertebrae of the upper cervical segment (occiput-atlas-axis) are firmly stabilized by numerous ligaments that permit physiological movement and deny or limit unwanted movements. These ligaments are the occipital-atlas-axis ligaments (Fig. 6–7), the transverse (cross) ligaments (Fig. 6–8), and the accessory atlanto-axial ligaments (Fig. 6–9).

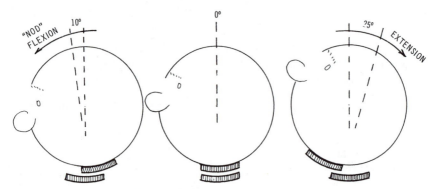

Figure 6–3. Occipital atlas movement.

The occiput moves exclusively in flexion extension upon the bodies of the atlas (C-1). Flexion occurs in the range of 10° and extension 25° for a total of 35°. No lateral flexion or rotation occurs at this joint. (From Cailliet, R: Neck and Arm Pain, ed 3. FA Davis, Philadelphia, 1991, p 18, with permission.)

Movement of the upper cervical spinal segment is limited by the facet articulations and the ligaments, but movement between C-2 upon C-3 is mechanically limited by the tip of the upper articular process of C-3 imping-ing upon the lateral margin of the vertebral foramen of C-2. The emergence of the greater superior occipital nerve (Fig. 6–10) is lateral to the atlas-axis membrane connecting the arches of the atlas and axis and innervates the fibrocartilaginous disc between their lateral bodies (Fig. 6–11). The mus-culature of the head and neck (Fig. 6–12) is related to possible headache and is either flexion of the head upon the neck and flexion of the neck (cervical spine) as well as extension of the head upon the neck and extension

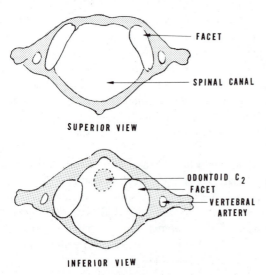

Figure 6–4. Atlas: First cervical vertebra.

The atlas (C-1) is viewed from above and below. The superior surface facets of the lateral bodies of the atlas artic-ulate with the condyles of the occiput. The inferior facets articulate with the superior fac-ets of the axis (C-2).

The site of the odontoid and the foramina of the vertebral arteries are depicted.

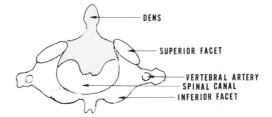

Figure 6–5. Axis: Second cervical vertebra.

The axis (C-2) is the second vertebra. The superior facets articulate as a synarthrosis with the inferior facets of the atlas (C-1). The inferior facets articulate with the superior facets of the third vertebra (C-3). The odontoid process (dens) ascends within the spinal canal of the atlas. It is held firmly against the anterior ramus by the transverse ligament.

of the cervical spine. There are also numerous small intrinsic muscles that rotate and laterally flex the neck.

Head pain has been attributed to dysfunction of the suboccipital muscles as well as the cervical spine muscles that attach to the head. These have been listed as sites of myofascial referred pain, which will be discussed in Chapter 7. Suffice here to say that head pain can be caused by muscles afflicted in poor posture, faulty movement of the head, posttrauma from hyperextension-hyperflexion injuries, or emotional tension. The implicated muscles are determined by knowledge of functional muscle anatomy, palpable tenderness of the afflicted muscles that refer to the head.[11]

The facet (zygapophyseal) joints are also innervated by segmental nerve roots, and they have been shown to refer pain to the occiput when injected

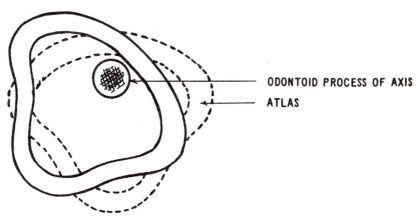

Figure 6–6. Rotation of the atlas upon the axis.

The atlas (C-1) rotates about the odontoid process of the axis (C-2) approximately 45° in each direction. (From Cailliet, R: Neck and Arm Pain, ed 3. FA Davis, Philadelphia, 1991, p 19, with permission.)

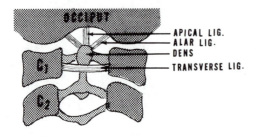

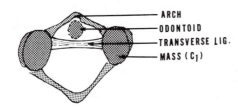

APICAL LIG.
ALAR LIG.
DENS
TRANSVERSE LIG.

ARCH
ODONTOID
TRANSVERSE LIG.
MASS (C₁)

Figure 6–7. Occipital-atlas-axis ligaments.

The apical and alar ligaments connect the tip of the dens with the occiput and limit lateral, anterior-posterior movement. They are considered also to restrict a degree of rotation.

The transverse ligament acts as a sling holding the dens against the anterior arch of the atlas (lower figure). It allows rotation of the dens but protects the cord within the spinal canal. (From Cailliet, R: Neck and Arm Pain, ed 3. FA Davis, Philadelphia, 1991, p 20, with permission.)

Figure 6–8. Transverse (cross) ligament.

The transverse ligament crosses the spinal canal and supports the dens against the anterior arch of the atlas. It sends a ligamentous portion superiorly to the foramen magnum and inferiorly to attach to the axis. (From Cailliet, R: Neck and Arm Pain, ed 3. FA Davis, Philadelphia, 1991, p 21, with permission.)

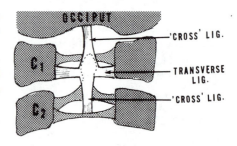

'CROSS' LIG.

TRANSVERSE LIG.

'CROSS' LIG.

ACESSORY LIG.

AXIS "BODY"

Figure 6–9. Accessory atlanto-axial ligaments.

The accessory atlanto-axial ligaments attach from the medial aspects of the bodies of the atlas (C-1) and descend in a converging direction to attach upon the body of the axis posterior to the odontoid process. (From Cailliet, R: Neck and Arm Pain, ed 3. FA Davis, Philadelphia, 1991, p 21, with permission.)

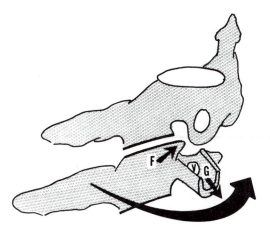

Figure 6–10. Mechanical limitation of rotation of the atlas upon the axis.

Rotation of the atlas upon the axis is limited by a mechanical locking in which the anterior tip of the upper articular process (F) impinges upon the lateral margin of the foramen on the vertebral artery (v). The nerve root of C-3 emerges through the gutter of C-3 (G).

and the capsule when distended.[12] These areas of referred pain have been documented (Fig. 6–13).

The dermatomal areas of cervical nerve roots have been well documented in the literature. The dermatomal area of reference of the upper three cervical nerve roots are depicted in Fig. 6–14. It is apparent that head pain from the cervical spine must emanate from the upper cervical regions, the occiput-atlas-axis.

CERVICOGENIC HEADACHE SYMPTOMATOLOGY

There is no specific characteristic of craniocervical headache because the etiology and tissue site remain unclear. Only by being associated with cervical movements or positions can the headache be considered cervicogenic.

Factors associated with craniocervical headache include the following:

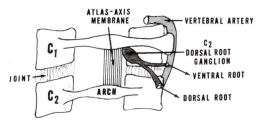

Figure 6–11. Emergence of the C-2 nerve root.

The C-2 dorsal ganglion lies under the obliquus inferior muscle (not shown) passing over the lateral atlanto-axial articulation. The C-2 nerve emerges lateral to the posterior atlas-axial membrane but does not penetrate it. It proceeds laterally to divide into a dorsal and ventral root. Its relationship to the vertebral artery is noted.

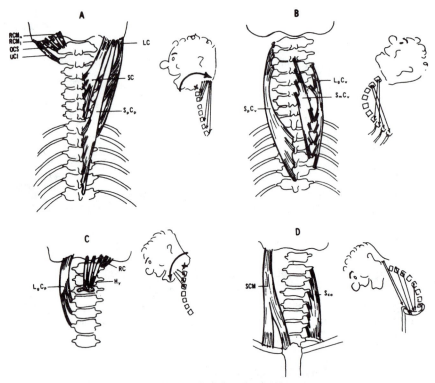

Figure 6–12. Musculature of the head and neck.

(A) and (B) The musculature of the extensor mechanism of the head and neck. (A) The capital extensors attach to the skull and move the head upon the neck. (B) The cervical extensors originate and attach upon the cervical spine and alter the curvature of the cervical spine. (C) and (D) Flexion musculature. (C) The capital flexors flex the head upon the neck. (D) The cervical flexors attach exclusively upon cervical vertebrae and have no significant functional attachment to the skull.

RCM_n	= rectus capitis minor		LC	= longissimus capitis
RCM_j	= rectus capitis major		SC	= semispinalis capitis
OCS	= obliquus capitis superior		S_pC_p	= splenius capitis
OCI	= obliquus capitis inferior		S_pC_v	= splenius cervicis
L_gC_p	= longus capitis		L_mC_v	= longissimus cervicis
RC	= rectus capitis anterior and lateral		S_mC_v	= semispinalis cervicis
H_y	= hyoideus and suprahyoid muscles		SCM	= sternocleidomastoid
			S_{ca}	= scalene medius and anticus

(From Cailliet, R: Neck and Arm Pain. ed 3. FA Davis, Philadelphia, 1991, p 23, with permission.)

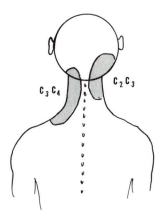

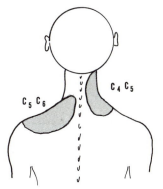

Figure 6–13. Referred areas of pain from invasion of the cervical zygapophyseal joints.

Experimental invasion of the zygapophyseal joints of the cervical spine refer symptoms into the areas of the head and neck as depicted.

1. Headache pain is chronic and relapsing in nature.

2. There are other painful disabling symptoms attributable to the cervical spine such as shoulder pain, interscapular pain, etc.

3. There is frequently a history of minor or major trauma.

4. Pain is related to movement of the head and neck as well as sustained postural positions.

5. Pain may start in the early morning and be attributed to a faulty sleeping position.

6. Headache is asymmetrical, not unilateral, and frequently radiates from the neck and base of the skull into the temporal or frontal area of the head. There is no precise site that ascertains the headache as being cervicogenic in comparison to other common types of headaches

Generally, this type of headache is stated to be a sensation of pressure and is diffuse. It is not, by definition, a throbbing headache. Cervicogenic headache has also been associated with symptoms of vertigo and dizziness

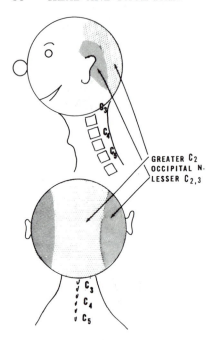

GREATER C₂
OCCIPITAL N.
LESSER C₂,₃

Figure 6–14. Dermatomal regions of the cervical nerves.

The areas depicted are the dermatomal areas of all the cervical nerves from C-2 to C-5 wherein C-2 and C-3 form the greater and lesser occipital nerves.

precipitated by neck and head movements. These are considered to be autonomic disturbances.[13]

There may be ipsilateral conjunctival injection, lacrimation, and lid edema but never a Horner's syndrome as is found in cluster headaches. There may be migrainelike symptoms such as nausea, phonophobia, photophobia, and even blurred vision, but the remainder of the symptom complex dispells the diagnosis of migraine or migraine variant.

The diagnosis of cervicogenic headache must include the reproduction of the symptoms from cervical maneuvers elicited during the history and examination or benefit from treatment to the cervical spine. To repeat, the cervical site must be the upper cervical (occiput-atlas-axis) region.

During the examination a specific cervical site must be evoked, not merely a generalized neck movement.[14,15] The specific segment can thus be revealed.[16]

Radiological changes are, unfortunately, difficult to relate to specific pathology unless they are structurally visible and clinically related to the physical examination. Dynamic (functional) x-rays are possibly more diagnostic than static films. CT scanning and MRI are better for viewing the upper cervical segments and their soft tissues than x-rays, but again they must correlate with the clinical evaluation.

HISTORY CONSISTENT WITH DIAGNOSIS OF CERVICOGENIC HEADACHE

In ascertaining the pathomechanics that would lead to a diagnosis of cervicogenic headache, some activity of or to the upper cervical spinal segment must be elicited. "Trauma"—either minor or major—may have been involved. Trauma implies irritation of the nociceptors in the tissues within the upper cervical segment: occiput-atlas-axis and their segmental nerve roots.

Minor trauma may be elicited in abnormal posture (Fig. 6–15) either in activities of everyday living[17] or in everyday occupational activities. The wearing of bifocal glasses can initiate a forward head posture with extension (elevation), increasing the cervical lordosis to ensure accurate vision (Fig. 6–16). That forward head posture in the seated position held for a prolonged period of time and aggravated by the intensity of the activity may initiate a headache (Fig. 6–17).

The trauma may be significant to severe and usually results from external impact such as a vehicular accident, sports injury, or a physical impact. The head undergoes hyperflexion or hyperextension (Fig. 6–18), meaning that the extent of flexion or extension exceeds the normal limits of the head and neck afforded by the ligaments, joint capsules, and muscles.

In the lower cervical segments (C-3 to C-7) the vertebrae that normally flex and extend with closing and opening of the intervertebral foramina (Fig. 6–19) exceed their physiological limits. The extensor and flexor cervical muscles undergo excessive and abrupt elongation, often overwhelming the contracted tone of the muscles (Fig. 6–20). There is reflex muscle "spasm" in addition to traumatized muscle tissue. Nociceptor tissue metabolites are released and pain results as well as limitation from the injured soft tissues. Myofascial pain results.

If the head at the moment of impact is rotated the head moves in a flexed (extended) lateral rotated manner, which not only causes excessive elongation of the ligaments, joint capsule, and muscles but also acutely narrows the foramina: the intervertebral and spinal canal (Fig. 6–21). The neural contents of the foramina undergo acute compression (Fig. 6–22) with possible resultant pain, hypoalgesia, or paresthesia.

In an abrupt overwhelming rear impact the head initially extends upon the cervical spine at the occipital cervical junction (Fig. 6–23) before the remainder of the cervical spine extends.

Because of the powerful ligamentous restraints of the occipital-atlas-axis joints (see Figs. 6–7, 6–8, 6–9) any passive motion of these joints must occur at the lateral body articulations, especially between atlas and axis (C-1 and C-2) causing subluxation of these joints. The dorsal root ganglia of cervical nerve C-2 carries sensation to the head via the greater superior occipital

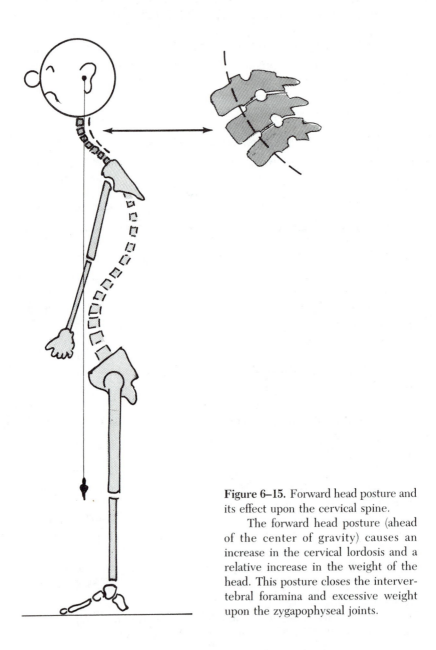

Figure 6–15. Forward head posture and its effect upon the cervical spine.

The forward head posture (ahead of the center of gravity) causes an increase in the cervical lordosis and a relative increase in the weight of the head. This posture closes the intervertebral foramina and excessive weight upon the zygapophyseal joints.

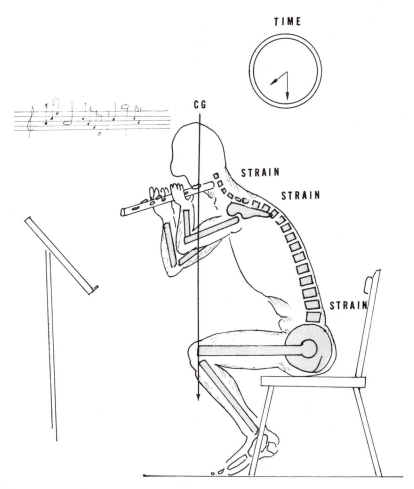

Figure 6–16. Faulty sitting postural effect upon the cervical spine.

In this person a forward head posture has been held for long periods of time and with intensity of attention. The effect is stressful and damaging to the tissues of the cervical spine. (From Cailliet, R: Abnormalities of Postures of Musicians. Vol 5, No 4, Medical Problems of Performing Artists. Hanley & Belfus, Philadelphia, 1990.)

AVOID

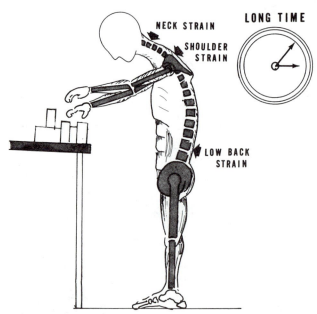

Figure 6–17. Faulty occupational standing posture.
Faulty standing posture creates occupational cervical stress. (From Cailliet, R: Neck and Arm Pain, ed 3. FA Davis, Philadelphia, 1991, p 79, with permission.)

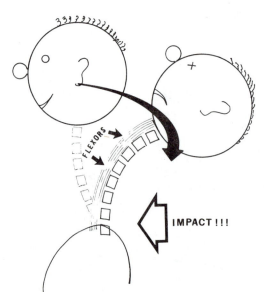

Figure 6–18. Occipital cervical hyperextension from external impact.

With a forceful impact the head and neck hyperextend causing injury to the neck flexors: the occipital-cervical and the cervical flexor muscles.

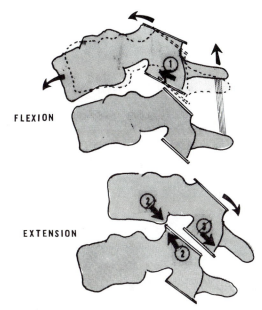

FLEXION

EXTENSION

Figure 6–19. Physiological flexion and extension of a lower cervical functional unit.
    Lower vertical units from C-3 to C-7. In flexion the facets (1) glide upon each other and the intervertebral foramina open.
    In extension the posterior aspect of the vertebral body (2) impinges and stops further extension. The facets glide backward (3) and the foramina narrow.

nerve (Fig. 6–24). Headache can result: a true postinjury craniocervicogenic headache.
    The "protective" resultant muscle spasm of the craniocervical muscles and their attachment to the occiput (Fig. 6–25) also contribute to the muscular response in hyperflexion-hyperextension injury headache.

DIAGNOSIS BASED ON RESPONSE
TO THERAPY

    These actions may be both diagnostic and therapeutic for cervicogenic headache.

    1. Manipulation of a specific segment of the head and neck, especially occipital-cervical manipulation. Here it must be noted, however, that the muscles are also "manipulated" and the headache may be a referred myogenic pain with involvement of a trigger point.
    2. Traction of the cervical spine which elongates the neck and distracts the joints as well as elongating the upper cervical and lower cervical muscles.
    3. Exercises to the neck, which may also improve range of motion,

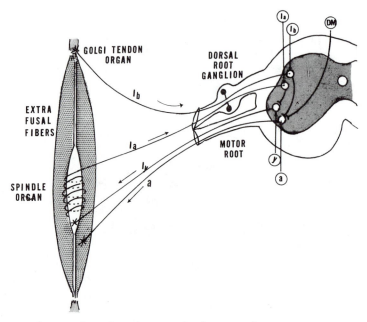

Figure 6–20. Neurological mechanism of reflex muscular spasm.

The extrafusal muscle fibers are kept at a specific length and tonus by a neural circuit effected by the spindle organs and tendon (Golgi) organs. Afferent impulses from these organs enter the dorsal column Ia and Ib, which has a neural contact with the anterior horn cells *(a)* and *(y)*. These nuclei innervate the extrafusal muscle fibers via the *y* and *a* fibers to initiate an appropriate contraction or sustained tone. All afferent fibers have their nuclei in the dorsal root ganglia.

separate the zygapophyseal joints, and diminish the sensitivity of trigger zones.

4. Local nerve blocks of the rami emerging from the occipital-atlanto and atlanto-axial joint spaces.[18–20]

5. Local injections of cervical muscles, which may eliminate the trigger areas.

6. Immobilization of the neck by a collar or brace with relief.

7. Local modalities such as ice, ultrasound, electrical stimulation, TENS, etc. to a specific segment of the cervical spine with relief. These modalities are also discussed in Chapter 10 but need to be emphasized in the treatment of cervicogenic headache.

8. Improvement of postures assumed during activities of daily living (ADL).

All the modalities and techniques of physical therapy to and for the cervical spine are thoroughly discussed and illustrated in Chapter 10 and

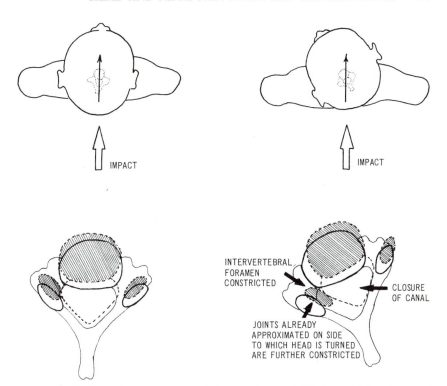

Figure 6–21. Hyperflexion-extension injury to the cervical spine with head rotated.

(A) The impact upon the head in a forward direction causes a to-and-fro flexion-extension resulting in symmetrical closing of the foramina and canal.

(B) With the head turned, there is constriction of the intervertebral foramen on the side toward which the head is rotated. This occurs physiologically but with impact is excessive. The spinal canal undergoes deformation with possible cord compression.

will not be discussed here. The same principles and techniques apply both in myofascial diseases and cervicogenic headache.

A recent review article attempting to relate chronic neck pain to cervicogenic headache fails to clarify the etiological relationship any more clearly than a review of the literature and personal clinical experience.[20] This article does highlight the fact that post-traumatic headaches are influenced by many nonmedical issues.[21]

A relationship of vascular hemicranial headache attributable to C-2 nerve root compression has been offered where headaches were diagnosed as vasoactive when local anesthetic injections temporarily relieved the head pain.[22] Complete permanent relief was attained by surgical decompression of the nerve root and ganglion of C-2.

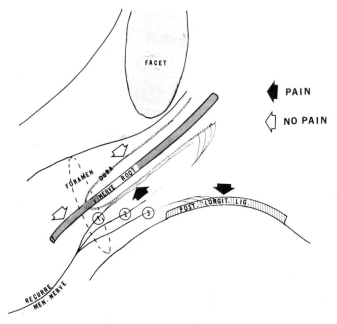

Figure 6–22. Compression effects upon neural contents of intervertebral foramen. .
    The black arrows indicate which fibers result in pain when compressed or trau-
matized. The white arrows indicate where compression does not result in pain.
    (1), (2), and (3) indicate the branching of the recurrent nerve of Luschka (meningeal
nerve) which carries somatic and sympathetic fibers.
    The foramen is located between the vertebral body (disk) and the posterior facet.

HEAD PAIN FROM THE LOWER
CERVICAL SPINE

    The emphasis has been on headache resulting from a "neuralgia" of the
C-1 and C-2 nerve roots but the role of the C-3 nerve has remained obscure.[23]
The C-3 dorsal ramus has a communicating branch to the greater occipital
nerve and proceeds as the third cervical nerve (C-3). This nerve supplies
the skin near the midline of the uppermost neck immediately below the
external occipital protruberance. Headaches attributed to this nerve root
have been eliminated by nerve blocks.
    That the cervicocranial junction can be responsible for headache is
evident from the literature on anomalies of this junction. These include
basilar invasion, congenital atlanto-axial dislocation, separate odontoid process, and occipitalization of the atlas. Lesions here such as tumors, Pott's
disease, Paget's disease, osteomyelitis, and rheumatoid arthritis have also
been implicated in headache. Their presence as diagnosed by radiological
and clinical findings clarify the relationship.[24]

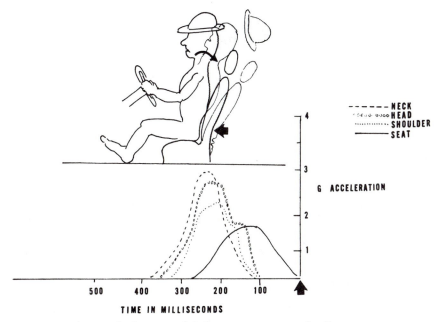

Figure 6–23. Upper body–cervical deformation in rear-end collisions.

With a force from behind, the head, neck, and shoulders deform at different points in time—all happens in less than 0.5 s. (From Cailliet, R: Neck and Arm Pain, ed 3. FA Davis, Philadelphia, 1991, p 88, with permission.)

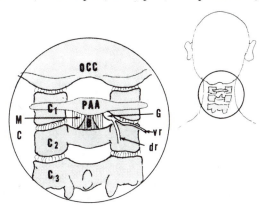

Figure 6–24. Cervical spine site of emergence of second nerve root (C-2).

The second cervical nerve emerges over the lateral bodies of atlas (C-1) and axis (C-2) and lateral to the atlas-axis membrane (M). The membrane attaches from the anterior arch. The posterior arch (PAA) is shown. The dens (D) of the axis (C-2) is depicted.

The nerve root (C-2) is shown with its ganglion (G) and ultimate division into a ventral branch (vr) and dorsal branch (dr). The C-2 nerve ultimately forms the greater superior occipital nerve. The "disk" is supplied by a twig of the dorsal branch. The occiput (OCC) and the cervical spine (C) are shown in the right figure.

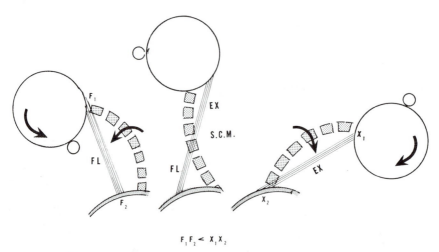

$$F_1 F_2 < X_1 X_2$$

Figure 6–25. Schematic: Muscle response to hyperflexion-extension injury of the cervical spine.

The middle figure indicates the sternocleidomastoid muscle (SCM) to be both a flexor muscle (FL) in its lower half and an extensor muscle (EX) in the upper half.

In the left figure the spine is hyperflexed, causing the SCM muscle to shorten and be totally a flexor muscle (FL) from points F_1 to F_2. In the rebound extension (right figure) the SCM muscle is now posterior to the lordosis and acts as an extensor (EX) with length X_1 to X_2.

The spindle system of this muscle is dissociated (uncoordinated) and trauma occurs to the shortened muscle being acutely extended (or vice versa).

There is little mention in the literature of head pain originating from the lower cervical spine. Brain observed that headache may be associated with a disc lesion at any cervical level but also claimed that the disc lesion was not the cause of the pain.[25] The basis for this latter statement was unsubstantiated in the article.

Raney and Raney[30] observed headache and facial pain in patients having cervical spondylosis based merely on radiological studies. The fact that headache was ameliorated in patients undergoing anterior interbody fusion of the cervical spine was reported.[26-28] Cloward, however, forcefully injected cervical discs with saline to reduce pain; this resulted in referred pain to the neck, shoulder, and interscapular area but no headache.[29]

The conclusion, currently, is that headache occurring from cervical spine disease is probably mediated by the paraspinous cervical muscles that occur reflexly from the noxious irritation of the cervical tissues through the sinu vertebral nerve (Fig. 6–26). The benefit from nerve blocks and epidural anesthesia (Fig. 6–27) also add to this speculation.

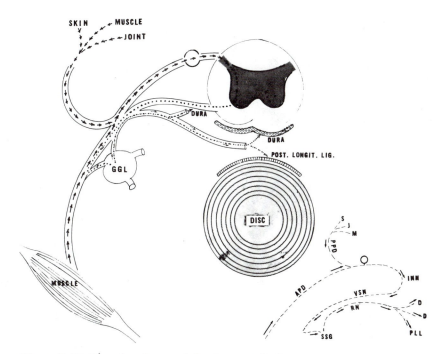

Figure 6–26. Neural pathways of the sinu vertebral nerve.

    The nerve pathways that initiate muscle spasm have been discussed in the text. The pathways are depicted in the right lower figure:

APD = anterior primary division
PPD = posterior primary division
S   = skin
J   = joint capsule
M   = extensor muscles
INN   = internuncial neurone
SSG = sensory spinal ganglion
RN   = recurrent meningeal nerve (sinu vertebral)
VSN = ventral spinal nerve
D   = dermatome
PLL = posterior longitudinal ligament
GGL = dorsal root ganglion

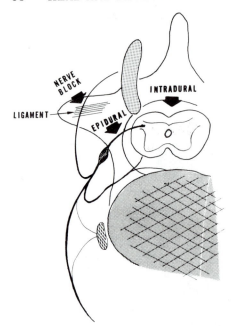

Figure 6–27. Mechanisms of nerve blocks and epidural injections.

The sites of therapeutic injections involve interruption of the nerve pathways indicated in the illustration.

REFERENCES

1. Berger, M and Gerstenbrand, F: Cervicogenic headache. In Rose, FC (ed): Handbook of Cinical Neurology, Vol 4: Headache. Elsevier, Amsterdam, 1986, pp 405–411.
2. Ad Hoc Committee on Classification of Headache: Classification of headache. Arch Neurol 6:173–176, 1962.
3. Williams, HL and Elkins, EG: Myalgia of the head. Arch Phys Therap 23:14–22, 1942.
4. Wolff, HG: Wolff's Headache and Other Head Pain, ed 3 rev. Oxford University Press, Oxford, 1972, pp 549–554.
5. Cailliet, R: Neck and Arm Pain, ed 3. FA Davis, Philadelphia, 1991, pp 147–164.
6. Friedenberg, ZB, Edeiken, J, Spencer, HN, and Tolentino, S: Degenerative transformation of the cervical spine. J Bone Joint Surg 41:61–70, 1959.
7. Bartschi-Rochaix, W: Headache of cervical origin. In Vinken, PJ and Bruyn, GW (eds): Handbook of Clinical Neurology, Vol 5. North-Holland Publishing, Amsterdam, 1983, pp 192–203.
8. Barré, JA: Sur un syndrome sympathetique cervical posterieur et sa cause fréquente, l'arthrite cervicale. Rev Neurol 33:1246–1248, 1926.
9. Sjaastad, O: Cervicogenic headache: An hypothesis. Cephalalgia 3:249–256, 1983.
10. Bogduk, N: Local anesthetic blocks of the second application in occipital headache. Cephalalgia 1:41–50, 1981.
11. Travell, JG and Simons, DG: Myofascial Pain and Dysfunction: The Trigger Point Manual. Williams & Wilkins, Baltimore, 1983, pp 290–294.
12. Bogduk, N and Marsland, A: The cervical zygapophyseal joints as a source of neck pain. Spine 13(6):610, 1988.
13. Hovelacque, A: Anatomie des nerfs craniens et rachdiens et du systeme grand sympathique, Vol 1. Paris, 1927, pp 873.
14. Maigne, R: Diagnostic et traitment des douleurs communes d'origine rachidienne: Une nouvelle approche. Expansion Scientifique Francaise, Paris, 1989, pp 342–346.

15. Nwuga, VC: Manipulation of the Spine. Williams & Wilkins, Baltimore, 1976, pp 47–56.
16. Berger, M: Neuroorthopadische Diagnostik und Therapieeffekte bei cervicalen Rotations-storungen. In Berger, M, Gerstenbrand, F, and Lewit, K (eds): Schmerz und Bewegungs-sytem. Gustav Fischer Verlag, Stuttgart, 1984, pp 163–172.
17. Cailliet, R: Neck and Arm Pain. FA Davis, Philadelphia, 1991, pp 43–58.
18. Busche, E and Wilson, PR: Atlanto-occipital and atlanto-axial injections in the treatment of headache and neck pain. Reg Anesth 14 (Suppl 2):45–48, 1989.
19. Ehni, G and Benner, B: Occipital neuralgia and the C1–2 arthrosis syndrome. J Neurosurg 61:961–965, 1984.
20. Wilson, PR: Chronic neck pain and cervicogenic headache. J Pain 7(1):5–11, 1991.
21. NcNamara, RM, O'Brien, MC, and Davidheiser, S: Posttraumatic neck pain: A prospective and follow-up study. Ann Emerg Med 17:906–911, 1988.
22. Jansen, J, Bardosi, A, Hildebrandt, J, and Lucke, A. Cervicogenic, hemicranial attacks associated with vascular irritation or compression of the cervical nerve root C2: Clinical manifestations and morphological findings. Pain 39:203–212, 1989.
23. Bogduk, N and Marsland, A: On the concept of third occipital headache. J Neurol Neurosurg Psychiat 49:775–780, 1986.
24. Edmeads, J: The cervical spine and headache. Neurol 38:1874–1878, December, 1988.
25. Brain, WR: Some unsolved problems of cervical spondylosis. Brit Med J 1:771–777, 1963.
26. Pawl, RP: Headache, cervical spondylosis and anterior cervical fusion. Surg Ann 9:391–408, 1977.
27. Peterson, DI, Austin, GM, and Dayes, A: Headache associated with discogenic disease of the cervical spine. Bull LA Neurol Soc 40:96–100, 1975.
28. White, AA, Southwick, WO, Deponte, RJ, Gainor, JW, and Hardy, R: Relief of pain by anterior cervical spine fusion for spondylosis. A report of 65 patients. J Bone Joint Surg 55:525, 1973.
29. Cloward, RB: The clinical significance of the sinuvertebral nerve of the cervical spine in relation to the cervical disc syndrome. J Neurol Neurosurg Psychiat 23:321–326, 1960.
30. Raney, AA and Raney, RB: Headache: A common symptom of cervical disc lesion. Arch Neurol 59:603–621, 1948.

CHAPTER 7

Myofascial Pain Syndromes

There are so many diagnostic terms applied to this syndrome and so many theories of pathomechanics that classification remains obscure. The relationship of face and head pain to fibromyalgia, as being primary or referred, also remains controversial, but this pain syndrome is so prevalent that it deserves thorough evaluation.

Terms used interchangeably include soft-tissue rheumatism, fibrositis, myofibrositis, fibromyositis, and fibromyalgia. All imply that the symptoms are the result of inflammation of the soft tissues, but the pathological lesions, the pathomechanics whereby this inflammation occurs, the significant diagnostic tests, and the meaningful therapeutic approach remain confusing.[1]

CLASSIFICATION AND IDENTIFICATION

The International Association for the Study of Pain (IASP) classifies these chronic musculoskeletal pain syndromes "without identifiable cause" as follows:[2]

1. Primary fibromyalgia syndrome (PFS) (also called fibrositis or diffuse myofascial pain syndrome; primary diffuse fibrositis syndrome)
2. Myosfascial pain syndrome (MPS) (also called specific myofascial pain syndrome)
3. Temporomandibular pain and dysfunction syndrome (TMPDS)

Of the accepted standardized diagnostic criteria, those of Yunus and associates are the most commonly accepted.[3] These criteria are as follows:

100

Obligatory

> • Generalized aches and pains or prominent stiffness, involving three or more anatomic sites for at least 3 months' duration
> • Absence of traumatic injury, structural rheumatic disease, infectious arthropathy, endocrine-related arthropathy, and abnormal laboratory tests

Major

> • Presence of three or more typical and consistent tender points

Minor

> • Symptoms modulated by physical activity
> • Symptoms altered by weather changes
> • Symptoms aggravated by anxiety or stress
> • Poor sleep
> • General fatigue or tiredness
> • Anxiety
> • Chronic headaches
> • Irritable bowel syndrome
> • Subjective swelling
> • Nonradicular and nondermatomal numbness

Whereas Yunus feels that 3 out of 10 minor criteria must be present, Wolfe disagrees, claiming that there must be 7 out of 14 tender points and the presence of generalized aches and pains.[4] Smythe, a pioneer in the subject of fibrositis, does not include psychological factors in diagnosing a clinical syndrome but relies exclusively upon "tender points" as major criteria.[5] Smythe's diagnostic criteria are as follows:

1. Widespread aching of more than 3 months' duration
2. Local tenderness at 12 of 14 specific sites
3. Skin roll tenderness over the upper scapular region
4. Disturbed sleep with morning fatigue and stiffness
5. Normal estimated sedimentation (ESR), serum glutamate oxaloacetate transaminase (SGOT), rheumatoid factor test, antinuclear factor (ANF), muscle enzymes, and sacroiliac films

While disallowing psychological factors Smythe described characteristic personality factors as being prone to this syndrome.[6]

Sleep disturbances, blandly espoused as diagnostic, were more scientifically correlated by Moldofsky.[7] He asserts that fibrositis syndromes mandate a specific sleep impairment before being considered, concluding that symptoms of chronic aching, nonrestorative sleep pattern with marked morning stiffness and fatigue, EEG findings of alpha intrusion in non-REM sleep, and localized tenderness of 12 or more of 14 specific sites are mandatory criteria for the diagnosis of fibrositis.[8]

McCain and Scudds cite these diagnostic criteria for myofascial pain syndrome:[9]

1. Local tenderness at one or a few points
2. A distinct pattern of referred pain
3. The presence of a taut, palpable band
4. A local twitch response to quick tapping
5. Associated muscle weakness and limited movement

As many, if not all, signs and symptoms are subjective or clinically "objective" based on a pertinent examination, all attempts to verify the neuromuscular diagnosis by electromyography (EMG) have failed.[10] There are, as yet, no specific EMG abnormalities claimed for fibromyositis (FS). FS is essentially a neuromuscular disorder without demonstrable electrodiagnostic findings.[11] The fatigue claimed by patients, however, has been substantiated electromyographically by Hagsberg and Kvarnstrom,[12] in which EMG fatigue changes occur in industrial neck and shoulder musculoskeletal pain.

A current study postulates that fibromyositis is akin to chronic fatigue syndrome and that both are depletion of the adrenogenic substance from prolonged stimulation of the posterior hypothalamus.[13] The prolonged stimulation is considered to result from prolonged stress, infection, immune disturbance, etc., which causes a sympathetic-parasympathetic imbalance. According to Cheu and Findley, the syndrome that results is similar to symptoms caused by continued use of reserpine medication. Further research is in the offing and may be reported by publication of this text.

Many clinicians, including the author, do not accept "absence of trauma" as an obligatory criterion for FS. Controversy has raged about the diagnosis of "traumatic fibromyositis." Trauma to muscles has shown amorphous mucoid substance between normal muscle fibers and fascicles.[11] Trauma leads to extravasation with release of serotonin. This in turn causes vasoconstriction and localized edema with release of histamine and heparin.[14] Postural trauma has been expounded by Travell and Simon.[15] The terms "tender points" and "trigger points" also do not enjoy unanimous agreement.[16]

It is apparent from the voluminous literature, exorbitant terminologies, varied criteria, controversial neuromusculoskeletal mechanisms, and pathological changes that the diagnosis falls into the wastebasket category, yet it presents as the primary complaint in most clinics, emergency centers, sports medicine clinics, and medicolegal cases.[17]

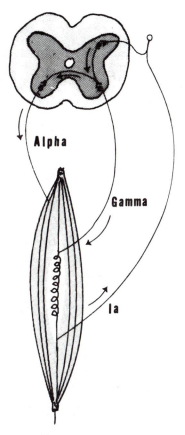

Figure 7–1. The spindle system.

The spindle system of the muscle moderates the tone of the extrafusal fibers. It transmits the information to the cord via Ia fibers at the cord level, where it modifies the tone of the extrafusal muscle fibers (innervated by somatic alpha fibers). The spindle system is "reset" to the appropriate tone via the gamma fibers. (From Cailliet, R: Neck and Arm Pain, ed 3. FA Davis, Philadelphia, 1991, p 114, with permission.)

SPINDLE SYSTEM

A mechanical neuromusculoskeletal concept of fibromyalgia can be postulated. "Trauma" of whatever type must be considered as causative. Physical trauma may be external trauma, mechanical trauma may be postural or sustained physical muscular stress, and psychological trauma may be tension, anxiety, anger, or stress. The initial neuromuscular dysfunction evolves into histological lesions within the musculoskeletal system that explain the subsequent symptoms.[18]

The dysfunction relates to inappropriate muscular contraction caused by the muscle spindles (Fig. 7–1), which are disorganized by "perturbers" (Fig. 7–2). Perturbers are factors that adversely influence the neuromuscular mechanisms which normally ensure smooth appropriate muscular coordination to perform the intended task. These factors influence the coordination centers of the central nervous system and are mediated via the afferent proprioceptive mechanoreceptive and nociceptive reflex activity emanating from the tendon organs (Golgi), the articular capsular mechanoreceptors and

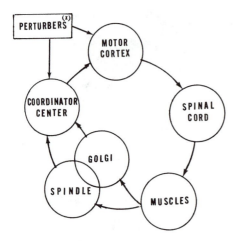

Figure 7–2. Perturber influence on neuromuscular mechanism.

The normal control of coordinated muscle activity is depicted in the design. Any intended activity requiring muscular activity is initiated in the motor cortex and follows the indicated sequence.

A perturber disturbs this normal flow. Among the many perturbers can be listed fatigue, anger, anxiety, compulsion, and depression as well as inappropriate training and practice.

proprioceptors, and the nociceptors mediated via C unmyelinated fibers. Common perturbers are fatigue, anger, impatience, anxiety, repression, boredom, tension, etc. Many organic diseases such as viral infections and hormonal imbalances as well as repeated microtraumata are also considered to be perturbers.

These perturbers interrupt or disrupt the normal coordination of the neuromuscular system, which in turn causes pain by damaging the peripheral tissues that have been inappropriately used in performing their function.

The reflex reaction from resultant soft-tissue pain is appreciated via the spinothalamic tracts (Fig. 7–3). The information ascending from the periphery is well documented (Fig. 7–4).[19]

The muscular contraction that is now "abnormal" from the perturber dissociation of the neurological mechanism imposes an acute stress (contraction or excessive elongation) upon the muscle that injures the sarcoplasmic reticulum. There results excessive release and retention of calcium ions from the excessive and prolonged muscular contraction. A review of normal muscular contraction will clarify the basis of abnormal contraction resulting in myositis.[20,21]

The muscles at rest and during physiological contraction and relaxation are under the voluntary control of the corticospinal system via the anterior horn cells within the cord gray matter. Their contraction, be it concentric or eccentric, is modulated by the spindle system (Fig. 7–5), which notifies the central nervous system that the act has been accomplished. It also modifies the rate of contraction or elongation as well as the force needed for the expected effort. The impulses from these spindle system afferents also enter the cord and ascend to the thalamus, the basal ganglia, and the cerebellum via the spinothalamic and spinocerebellar tracts. Coordination involves multiple neuromuscular systems all appropriately related (Fig. 7–2).

Should there be a violation of the forces expended upon or by the

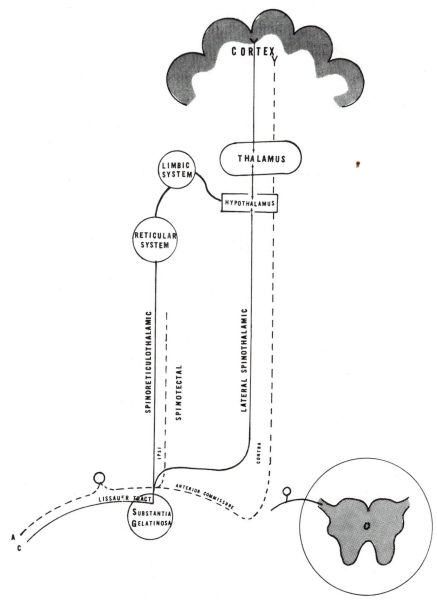

Figure 7–3. Two major neurophysiologic transmission systems.
Spinothalamocortical system (A) has spatiotemporal localization; spinoreticulothalamic system (C) has no localization but is involved in emotional (limbic) and avoidance reaction. (From Cailliet, R: Soft Tissue Pain and Disability, ed 2. FA Davis, Philadelphia, 1988, p 26, with permission.)

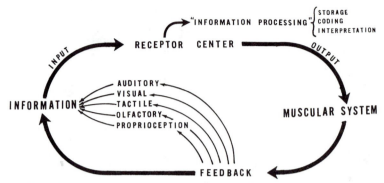

Figure 7–4. Information from internal and external environments via receptors is involved in the process of learning a skill.

Almost all behavior is motor in nature; humans respond with voluntary and involuntary movements, which include posture. The learning of skills proceeds in phases (see text). Feedback is one of the most important concepts in learning and is an important factor in the control of movement and behavior. (From Cailliet, R: Soft Tissue Pain and Disability, ed 2. FA Davis, Philadelphia, 1988, p 10, with permission.)

musculoskeletal system from any of the above-mentioned traumata the system becomes temporarily dysfunctional. Dependant upon the severity, duration, or recurrence of the stress of these perturbers, there is a commensurate muscular reaction.

Muscular contraction occurs by shortening of the contractile elements as a sliding of the actin filaments over the myosin filaments. This process occurs by virtue of depolarization from the calcium that is released from the sarcoplasmic reticulum. After the contraction the reticulum reaccumulates the calcium (Fig. 7–6).

If the contraction is excessive, excessive calcium is liberated and remains, causing the muscle to remain contracted. This sustained contraction causes uncontrolled excessive metabolism within the muscle; this in turn demands an extra vasomotor reaction. The metabolites liberated by this muscular contraction cause vasoconstriction. This neurovascular reaction has a retrograde sympathetic and somatic nervous system reaction wherein the muscle remains contracted. By remaining contracted the muscle remains excessively metabolically active, yet avascular.

There also occurs a depletion of adenosine triphosphate (ATP), which inhibits a release of the myosin filaments to disengage from the actin filaments, and the sarcomeres become rigid.[22]

The antagonist muscle should normally elongate at the precise degree as the agonist shortens. An excessive elongation of the antagonist muscle causes excessive elongation with trauma to the fascia as well as the muscle fiber bands (Fig. 7–7).

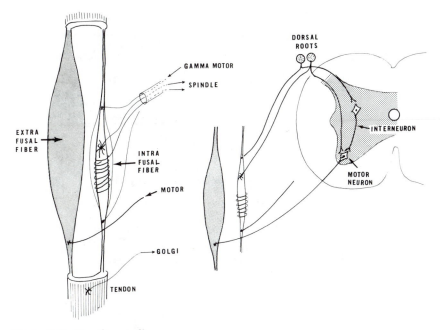

Figure 7–5. Muscle spindles.

The contractile fibers are known as extrafusal fibers and are innervated by the motor neuron. The intrafusal fibers contain the spindles which end in annulospiral fibers and flower-spray endings. These fibers send impulses to the cord, conveying stretch responses. In voluntary extrafusal contraction there is no stretch reflex. In an abrupt contraction of the extrafusal fibers, such as a tendon jerk, there is a reflex via the interneuron that stimulates the motor neuron. The tendon stretch is mediated through the Golgi tendon organ. The gamma motor fibers adjust the length and thus the response of the spindle system. (From Cailliet, R: Neck and Arm Pain, ed 3. FA Davis, Philadelphia, 1991, p 89, with permission.)

The blood supply to the muscle that is either elongated or excessively contracted by the shortened and sustained contracted muscle is diminished. This causes ischemia and an accumulation of the metabolic residue of muscular contraction—lactic acid. Traumata to the blood vessel causes liberation of serotonin from the liberated platelets; this in turn causes vasomotor contraction (Fig. 7–8) and further activates the muscular contraction. All these activities are unphysiological, releasing substances such as histamine, kinin, serotonin, and a breakdown of arachidonic acid (Fig. 7–9), which further breaks down to phospholipids, ultimately forming prostaglandins. At the site of muscle injury the extravasated blood releases platelets (the source of serotonin),[23] increases mast cells (a source of histamine),[24] fibroblasts, and initiates changes within the intercellular matrix (Fig. 7–10). Ischemia of muscle causes structural changes in the deprived muscle thus impairing

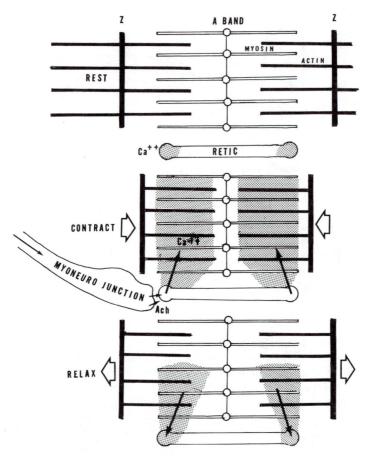

Figure 7–6. Muscle contraction.

The upper illustration depicts the muscle at rest. The actin filaments are attached to the Z line and maintain a parallel relationship to the myosin filaments which form an A band. The sarcoplasmic reticulum (retic) contains calcium ions that when released (middle figure) cause the actin and myosin filaments to glide together shortening the sarcomere. This is a muscle contraction.

The calcium ions return to the reticulum and allow the sacromere to resume its resting (relaxed) position.

The myoneural junction is the termination of the motor neuron axon that, when stimulated, releases acetylcholine (Ach) which increases the permeability of the muscle membrane causing an influx of sodium ions. This depolarizes the membrane causing calcium to flow resulting in a muscle contraction.

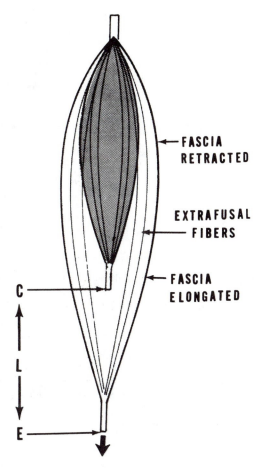

Figure 7–7. Fascial limits to muscular elongation.

Any muscle bundle can elongate to the extent that its fascial sheath permits. The extrafusal fibers elongate fully, but the fascia must be passively elongated. Fascial contracture restricts muscular elongation and joint range of motion. L = length, C = contracted, E = elongated. (From Cailliet, R: Neck and Arm Pain, ed 3. FA Davis, Philadelphia, 1991, p 115, with permission.)

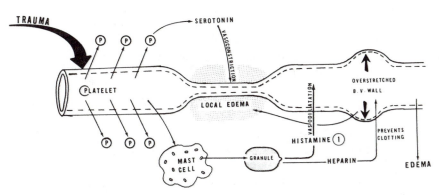

Figure 7–8. Schematic concept of the effect of trauma, a vasochemical reaction.

(From Cailliet, R: Soft Tissue Pain and Disability, ed 2. FA Davis, Philadelphia, 1988, p 31, with permission.)

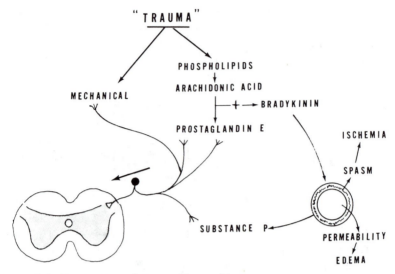

Figure 7–9. Nociceptive substances liberated by trauma.

Regardless of its type, trauma may be mechanical and liberate histamines and other noxious substances. Trauma may also break down phospholipids to become arachidonic acid, which forms prostaglandin E. This end substance reacts on the end membrane of the sensory nerve fibers, initiating the sensation ultimately interpreted as "pain."

Noxious substances liberated by trauma may also act on the blood vessels, causing "spasm" and may increase the permeability of these vessels, causing edema. (Modified from Brom, B: Neurobiological concepts of pain: Its assessment and therapy. In Brom, B (ed): Pain Measurements in Man: Neurophysiological Correlates of Pain. Elsevier Science Publishing, New York, 1984, p 18.)

function. These findings have been documented by muscle biopsies in patients considered to have sustained painful muscle contractions.[25]

These liberated chemicals are nociceptive that irritate end organs of C fibers resulting in pain from irritation of the spinothalamic tracts. The chemical reaction sustains the neuromuscular contracture that initially was autonomic via the spindle system.

The articulations influenced by the contracture of muscles—agonist or antagonist—are also violated with a synovial reaction (inflammation) which accentuates the nociceptor activity. The proprioceptors of the synovial joints also emit impulses via the proprioceptor system (Fig. 7–11). All these factors and possibly others explain the dysfunction—initially neuromuscular with resultant pain and shortening ("stiffness")—that impairs the patient. The secondary musculoskeletal reactions account for the pain and the presence of fiber bands and even the nodular triggers (Fig. 7–12). The sustained contraction of muscle in the region of the band causes further vascular damage, with release of more serotonin (a vasoconstrictor), histamine (a

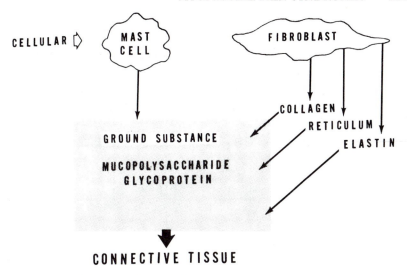

Figure 7–10. Cellular and chemical changes affecting connective tissue.
(From Cailliet, R: Soft Tissue Pain and Disability, ed 2. FA Davis, Philadelphia, 1988, p 4, with permission.)

vasodilator), kinins, and prostaglandins, which irritate the ending of sensory C fibers.

DIAGNOSIS

The diagnosis of myofascial pain as it affects the face and head must be based mostly on history as the clinical findings are sparse and the laboratory confirmation is essentially negative.

To diagnose an active myofascial trigger point there must be an ascertainable history of trauma (either a micro or macro injury), inappropriate muscular activity, or muscular overactivity. From the history there must follow objective evidence of abnormal muscular function in which the involved muscle cannot resume resting length and is painful and tender. The involved muscle may be weak and, when stretched, is limited in its passive extension to its expected normal resting length. The affected muscle must be a palpable taut band of tender muscle. The tenderness may be "exquisite" as elicited by digital pressure on the spot. Tender spots found within the skin or scars are considered to be nonmyofascial trigger points.

In determining that the patient's complaint of muscle tenderness within the head or face is a component of myofascial pain, specific points must be elicited elsewhere in the body characteristic of the syndrome.

Myofascial pain usually begins as an acute muscular pain and tenderness from a strain or sprain and is often attributed to muscle fatigue from an

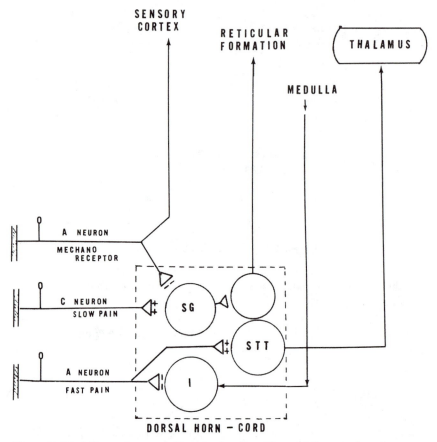

Figure 7–11. Afferent (sensory) fibers in the dorsal horn of the spinal cord.

Nociceptive stimuli are transmitted via three types of peripheral nerve axons: A beta (mechanoreceptors), C neurons (transmitting slow pain sensations), and A gamma (transmitting fast pain sensations). They synapse with fibers of the substantia gelatinosa (SG) and enkephalinergic interneuron (I) and ultimately ascend via the spinothalamic tract (STT) to the thalamus. There are numerous interconnections that ascend to the cortex via other routes and via the reticular system. (Modified from Bond, M: Pain: Its Nature, Analysis and Treatment, ed 2. Churchill Livingstone, Edinburgh, 1984, p 26.)

activity. The pain is characterized as deep and aching. Rarely, if ever, is it described as burning.

The involved muscle pain is aggravated by active contraction or stretch of that muscle. Tenderness is reasonably precisely localized and persistent in its site. Pain and tenderness appear to be accentuated by cold, damp weather, stress, fatigue, ancillary infections, etc. Pain, tenderness, and stiffness appear more marked upon arising in the morning and tend to recur after any inadvertent activity during the day.

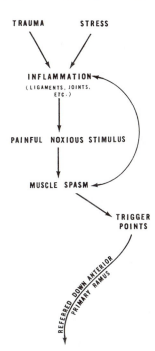

Figure 7–12. Schematic concept of pain manifestation.

Trauma to joints, ligaments, and other soft tissues ultimately creates trigger points that refer pain to distal sites. (From Cailliet, R: Soft Tissue Pain and Disability, ed 2. FA Davis, Philadelphia, 1988, p 32, with permission.)

Associated autonomic dysfunctional symptoms are frequent and may include excessive lacrimation, pilomotor activities, changes in sweating patterns, feeling of cold in the extremity, sleep disturbance, and evidence of depression.

Often the sequelae of muscular pain after trauma remain for long periods of time long after the initial incident is forgotten.[26] Pain may continue for months and even years and, even though considered benign, can be significantly debilitating.[27]

PHYSICAL EXAMINATION

The muscle that is to be examined must be stretched until its fibers are under tension. This stretch should evoke local discomfort but not referred pain. Pain is elicited when the involved muscle is stretched to two-thirds of its normal length. Palpation then is performed along the entire length of the muscle until the point of maximum tenderness is found. Persistent local pressure upon that site is maintained to confirm persistent tenderness. Often examination of a tender muscle is elicited by pressure upon the muscle with pressure imposed against the underlying bone, depending upon the site of the muscle. The muscle can actually be palpated in a squeezing manner between two examining fingers if the muscle belly is so accessible. Actively

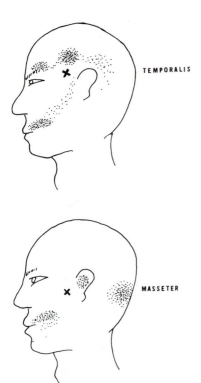

TEMPORALIS

MASSETER

Figure 7–13. Referred myofascial sites of pain in the head and face.

The dotted regions of the face and head indicate the sites of referral when the trigger (X) site is injected or irritated.

The upper illustration reveals the trigger site in the temporalis muscle and the lower drawing the trigger within the masseter muscle.

stretching the involved muscle intensifies the pain which reflexively causes further contraction as the irritable focus is intensified. This explains why daily activity often intensifies the localized muscle pain and tenderness.

When an involved muscle is rolled between two fingers there may be a muscular reaction termed as "twitch" or a "jump sign." If there is a nerve in the vicinity of the inflamed muscle there may result a neurologically referred pain or paresthesia such as distal numbness, tingling, hyperparesthesia or hyperesthesia.

There are zones or sites of referred myofascial pain which are important to elicit and recognize in evaluating head and face pain as emanating from myofascial trigger sites. Several prominent sites are illustrated in Figs. 7–13, 7–14, and 7–15.

The sites of predictable trigger points and their areas of referral have been well-documented by Travell and Rinzler.[28] In the illustrations, the dark cross is the site of the trigger from which emanates a referred pain area (shaded site). The darker areas are the common sites, whereas the lighter spotted areas are less common or merely occasional sites. The following criteria have been propounded for the diagnosis of an active myofascial trigger point and its referral pattern.[29]

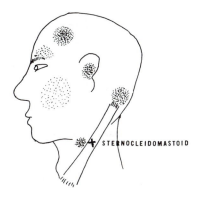

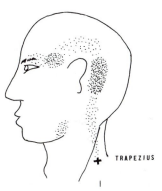

Figure 7–14. Referred patterns from trigger sites within the sternocleidomastoid and trapezius muscles.

The dotted areas are the referral sites when the trigger sites (X) are injected or irritated. The trigger sites here are within the sternocleidomastoid muscle (upper drawing) and the trapezius muscle (lower drawing).

    1. A history of sudden onset after an acute overload of stress or gradual onset with chronic overload of the affected muscle

    2. Characteristic patterns of pain that are referred from myofascial trigger points within specific individual muscles

    3. Weakness and restriction in the stretch range of motion of the affected muscle

    4. A taut palpable band in the affected muscle

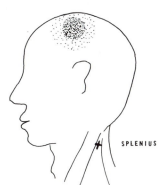

Figure 7–15. Referral zone of trigger site within the splenius muscle.

When the trigger site within the splenius muscle (X) is injected the referral site is experienced in the dotted area of the skull.

5. Exquisite focal tenderness to digital pressure in the band of taut muscle fibers

6. A local twitch response elicited through "snapping" palpation or needling of the tender spot

7. Reproduction of the patient's pain complaint by pressure on or needling of the tender spot

8. The elimination of symptoms by therapy directed specifically to the affected muscles

It is apparent that the clinician needs precise knowledge of muscle origin and insertion as well as function and that a diligent search for the trigger points must take place. Reproduction of the complaint confirms the diagnosis as evidenced in the above criteria. The common sites of trigger points and the areas of referral must be studied and elicited for accurate diagnosis.

LABORATORY CONFIRMATION

By definition all laboratory tests implying other rheumatological, endocrine, and neurological disease *must* be negative. Electromyographic examination of the trigger points have been reported as "abnormal," but none have specifically designated a precise pattern. More recently, thermography has been expounded as diagnostic as the areas over the trigger points have had an increase in skin temperature.[30] Autonomic dysfunction in the area justify changes evidenced on thermography, but again in a nonspecific manner.

TREATMENT

Management rather than treatment appears more appropriate as the condition is a benign disabling painful state that does not impair longevity or imply ominous sequelae or complications. The objective of treatment is to decrease the pain to tolerable levels, improve daily function, and prevent permanent physical and psychological disability.

Spraying and stretching the muscle bands or trigger points is considered the mainstay procedure once the diagnosis has been made. This approach deactivates the irritable tender spots and intercepts the neuromuscular patterns, even if there are widespread tender spots. It does not require precise localization of the trigger points but merely localizing the individual muscle involved. Local myoneural injection of the trigger point requires more precise localization.

Spray with a vasocoolant before and during stretching has been advocated.[31] The technique has been well documented: the muscle involved is sprayed in a direction away from its origin at a 30° angle for several sweeps of the vasocoolant spray until there is a slight frost on the skin above the muscle. The muscle is then stretched. After a treatment hot applications are indicated, but not active exercises.

Treatment of a trigger point with referral pattern implies direct injection of an anesthetic agent into the trigger point. This presumes carefully eliciting the specific trigger point before injection. Dry needling has been proposed, as has sterile saline,[32] but not found as effective as injection of a local anesthetic agent. The inclusion of steroids in the injection has its advocates but is not universally accepted as beneficial.

Treatment following spray and stretch may include deep heat, massage, TENS, biofeedback, and acupuncture if the pain is intractible or persistent. As the condition is mediated by neuromusculoskeletal factors, these should be identified (posture, occupational positions, stressful working patterns, psychosocial stress, etc.), and where tissue inflexibility is elicited, these tissues (muscle and its fascia) should be stretched actively and passively. Where there is weakness, incoordination, or muscular imbalance, appropriate exercises must be instituted. Aerobic exercises have proven valuable.[33]

A total body evaluation is mandatory as it is evident that patients with myofascial impairment have generalized imbalance of posture, activities of daily living, and the presence of many perturbers (Fig. 7–16).

Posture must be evaluated in standing and sitting positions, in daily activities of living, and during work. Duration of assumed posture must be corrected if excessive.[34] Frequent changes (60-second breaks) in assumed postures must be encouraged.[35] Daily stretch exercises must be prescribed, and the specific muscle group needing stretch must be specified. Aerobic exercises are finding strong advocacy. Good general reconditioning is beneficial for numerous reasons.

The anxiety, stress reaction, and depression—so prevalent in fibromyositis—must also be treated. Counseling and even psychotherapy may be needed. The term "tension" as a mental state that it is "all in the head" must be diffused and explained to the patient. Once the stressful situations are unearthed they must be corrected. Biofeedback is often of value, as is stress management.

Reassurance that the disease is benign—in fact, not even a disease—has been advocated by all who specialize in treating myofascial syndromes. A meaningful explanation of all the factors, procedures, and modalities must be given to the patient.

INFLUENCE OF THE SYMPATHETIC NERVOUS SYSTEM

Pain that originates by peripheral nociceptor impulses mediated via the unmyelinated C fibers is transmitted to the dorsal horn of the cord through

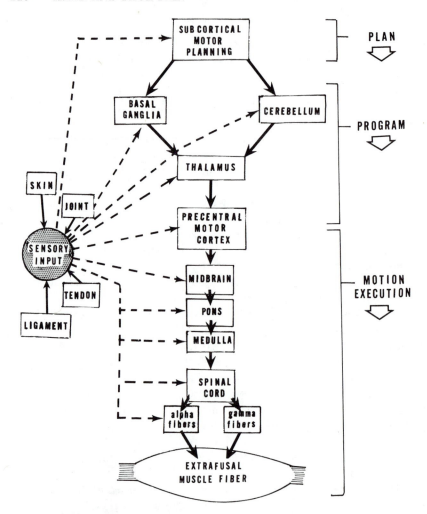

Figure 7–16. Spinal and supraspinal motor centers.
(Adapted from Schmidt, RF) (From Cailliet, R: Shoulder Pain, ed 3. FA Davis, Philadelphia, 1991, p 197, with permission.)

the dorsal root ganglion (Fig. 7–17). These impulses implicating the layers of Rexed I and II are termed the substantia gelatinosum. They enter the sensory nociceptive pool (Fig. 7–18) that progress via the lateral spino-thalamic tracts to the midbrain, thalamus, and hypothalamus ultimately to impact upon the cortical centers where pain is appreciated.

Whereas there is an implication of autonomous nervous system involve-ment in myofascial pain syndrome, there has not been significant reference to this in the literature. Recent studies have documented concepts explaining sympathetic maintained pain (SMP)[36] and also explained the sensitivity that

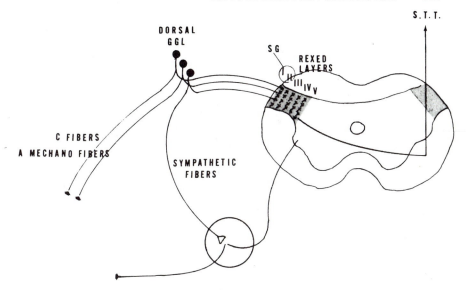

Figure 7–17. Causalgic (autonomic) transmission of pain sensation.

Trauma irritates somatic afferent C fibers, A mechanofibers, and sympathetic fibers, whose impulses proceed to the dorsal column of the cord. There is a cord interneuron connection that transmits efferent impulses via the autonomic system to the periphery, which sensitizes the skin to mechanical (light touch) input.

At the cord, the afferent fibers initiate neuronal activity in the Rexed layers of the dorsal column. The Rexed layers I and II are the substantia gelatinosa. (Modified from Roberts, WS: A hypothesis on the physiological basis for causalgia and related pains. Pain 24:297, 1986. From Cailliet, R: Soft Tissue Pain, ed 2. FA Davis, Philadelphia, 1988, with permission.)

results in the involved tissues (vasomotor changes and the nodularity noted in myofascial painful areas).

The initial impulses transmitted through the unmyelinated C fibers enter the dorsal columns (layers of Rexed) where they stimulate the nerve fibers of the wide dynamic neurones (WDN) and cause a hypersensitivity of that region (Fig. 7–19). A hypersensitivity may also be initiated in the traumatized area where involved nerves may be traumatized. An axonal outgrowth may result that secretes more norepinephrine, which in turn enhances the sympathetic nervous system reaction (Fig. 7–20). Mechanoreceptors in the periphery that normally transmit their impulse through the dorsal root ganglion to affect the layers of Rexed now impact upon the hypersensitive DN region, and pain results from what otherwise was a mechanosensation to touch and movement. A painful sensation (nociception) can now be initiated by mere touch, temperature change, or vibration.

Besides continuing centrally to the thalamic-hypothalamic neurones via the spinothalamic tracts, the WDN also have a neuronal attachment to the lateral horn cells that innervate the sympathetic structures (sweat glands,

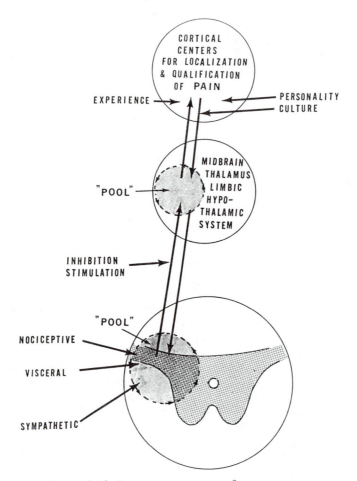

Figure 7–18. Sensory transmission of pain sensation.

blood vessels, hair follicles), causing the dystrophic changes in the peripherally involved area.

In relating this sympathetic nervous system to myofascial pain the following can be explained:[37,38]

1. Painful skin rolling
2. Hypersensitivity of the skin and muscles to touch or pressure
3. Vasomotor changes such as pallor, hyperemia, subjective coldness, hyperhydrosis, etc.
4. Marked reaction (thalamic, hypothalamic, etc.) to emotional stresses
5. Favorable response to antidepressants, beta blockers, etc.

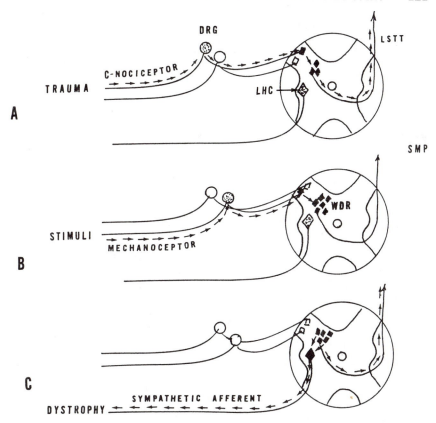

Figure 7–19. Postulated neurophysiologic mechanism of sympathetic maintained pain (SMP).

The transmission via C-nociceptor fibers *(A)* of impulses from the peripheral tissues that have been traumatized and created peripheral nociceptor chemicals (see details in text). These impulses pass through the dorsal root ganglion (DRG) to activate the gray matter of the cord in the Rexed layers. When sensitized, they are termed *wide dynamic range neurones* (WDR). The WDR, becoming very irritated, receive impulses from the periphery via the A-mechanoreceptor fibers, *(B)* which normally transmit sensations of touch, vibration, temperature, etc. When the periphery is stimulated (skin touch, pressure, or joint movement), these impulses enhance and maintain the irritability of the WDR. The impulses from the WDR continue cephalad though the lateral spinal thalamic tracts (LSTT) to the thalamic centers with resultant continued pain. The WDR impulses irritate the lateral horn cells (LHC), which generate sympathetic impulses that innervate the peripheral tissues resulting in the symptoms and findings of dystrophy *(C)*. (From Cailliet, R: Shoulder Pain, ed 3. FA Davis, Philadelphia, 1991, p 234, with permission.)

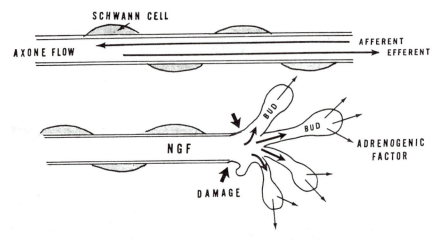

Figure 7–20. Axonal outgrowths forming a neuroma (schematic).

After a nerve injury with compression or partial to total severance, the nerve growth factor (NGF) stimulates the nerve to advance distally and form "buds," which create more endings than the normal nerve shown in the upper drawing.

By virtue of the greater secretion of adrenogenic factors, the nerve becomes more sensitive to adrenogenic agonists and transmits more potential pain fiber impulses to the spinal cord (see also Fig. 7–18). (From Cailliet, R: Shoulder Pain, ed 3. FA Davis, Philadelphia, 1991, p 231, with permission.)

Whereas the term "inflammation" is mentioned in the etiology of myofascial pain, nonsteroidal anti-inflammatory drugs have proven ineffectual.

Abnormal sleep patterns have been postulated as provocative and aggravating to myofascial patients. These abnormal sleep patterns must be controlled. Depression is also a major factor in this syndrome and must be addressed.[39] Both the nonrefreshing sleep and the depression can be addressed by the use of antidepressants. A recommended drug that has proven effective is a tricyclic, doxepin hydrochloride, 10 to 25 mg taken 1 hour before bedtime. This class of drug interferes with serotonin metabolism increasing the amine concentration within the central nervous system. Psychological help or psychiatric intervention may actually be needed if antidepressant medicine and supportive therapy fail.

REFERENCES

1. Buckelew, SP: Fibromyalgia: A rehabilitation approach. Am J Phys Med Rehabil 68(1):37–42, 1989.
2. International Association for the Study of Pain, Subcommittee of Taxonomy: Chronic pain syndromes and definition of pain terms. Pain (Suppl)3:S1–S225, 1986.
3. Yunus, MB, Masi, AT, Calabro, JJ, Miller, KA, and Feigenbaum, SL: Primary fibromyalgia

(fibrositis) clinical study of 50 patients with matched normal controls. Semin Arthritis Rheum 11:151–171, 1981.

4. Wolfe, F and Cathey, MA: Prevalence of primary and secondary fibrositis. J Rheumatol 10:965–968, 1983.

5. Smythe, HA: "Fibrositis" as a disorder of pain modulation. Clin Rheum Dis 5:823–832, 1979.

6. Smythe, HA: Nonarticular rheumatism and psychologenic musculoskeletal syndromes. In McCarty, D (ed): Arthritis and Allied Conditions. A Textbook of Rheumatology, ed 5. Lea & Febiger, Philadelphia, 1982, pp 1083–1094.

7. Moldofski, H: Sleep and musculoskeletal pain. Am J Med (Suppl 3A) 81:85–89, 1986.

8. Smythe, HA and Moldofski, H: Two contributions to understanding of the "fibrositis" syndrome. Bull Rheum Dis (Series No 1) 28:928–931, 1977–1978.

9. McCain, GA and Scudds, RA: The concept of primary fibromyalgia (fibrositis): Clinical value, relation and significance to other chronic musculoskeletal pain syndrome. Pain 33:273–287, 1988.

10. McBroom, F, Walsh, N, and Dumitru, D: Electromyography in primary fibromyalgia syndrome. Clin J Pain 4:117–119, 1988.

11. Awad, EA: Interstitial myofibrositis: Hypothesis of the mechanism. Arch Phys Med 54:449–453, 1974.

12. Hagsberg, M and Kvarnstrom, S: Muscular endurance and electromyographic fatigue in myofascial shoulder pain. Arch Phys Med Rehabil 65:522–525, 1984.

13. Cheu, JW and Findley, T: Integrated Parallel-Cycle Model of Chronic Fatigue Syndrome. University of Medicine and Dentistry, NJ: Personal correspondence, 1991.

14. Edvinsson, L, MacKenzie, ET, McCulloch, J, and Uddman, R: Nerve supply and receptor mechanism in intra- and extracerebral blood vessels. In Olesen, J and Edvinsson L, (eds): Basic Mechanisms of Headache. Elsevier, Amsterdam, 1988, pp 138–139.

15. Travell, JG and Simon, DG: Myofascial Pain and Dysfunction: The Trigger Point Manual. Williams & Wilkins, Baltimore, 1983, p 310.

16. Foster, JB: The clinical features of some miscellaneous neuromuscular disorders. In Walton, JN (ed): Disorders of Voluntary Muscle, ed 3. Churchill Livingstone, Edinburgh, 1974, pp 898–899.

17. Thompson, JM: Tension Myalgia as a Diagnosis at the Mayo Clinic and Its Relationship to Fibrositis, Fibromyalgia and Myofascial Pain Syndrome. Mayo Clin Proc 65:1237–1248, 1990.

18. De Vries, HA: Physiology of Exercise, ed 3. WC Brown, Dubuque, IA, 1966, pp 473–485.

19. Campbell, HJ: Correlative Physiology of the Nervous System. Academic Press, New York, 1965, pp 99–107.

20. McMahon, TA: Muscles, Reflexes and Locomotion. Princeton University Press, Princeton, NJ, 1984, pp 53–84.

21. Wolfe, F, Simons, D, Fricton, J, Bennett, RM, Goldenberg, DL, Gerwin, RD, Hathaway, D, McCain, GA, Russell, IJ, Sanders, H, and Skootsky, S: The fibromyalgia and myofascial pain syndromes: A study of tender points and trigger points in persons with fibromyalgia, myofascial pain syndrome and no disease (abstr). Clin J Pain 7(1):45, 1991.

22. Miehlke, K, Schulze, G, and Eger, W: Klinische und experimentelle Untersuchungen zum Fibrositis-syndrome. Z Rheumatorsch 19:310–330, 1960.

23. Hillis, LD and Lange, RA: Serotonin and acute ischemic heart disease. N Engl J Med 324(10):668–689, 1991.

24. Stenger, RJ, Spiro, D, Scully, RE, and Shannon, JM: Ultrastructural and physiologic alterations in ischemic skeletal muscle. Am J Pathol 40:1–20, 1962.

25. Fassbender, HG and Wegner, K: Morphologie und Pathogenese des Weichteilrheumatismus. Z Rheumatorsch 32:355, 1973.

26. Elson, LM: The jolt syndrome: Muscle dysfunction following low-velocity impact. Pain Management Nov–Dec:317–326, 1990.
27. Ingle, JI and Beveridge, EE: Endodontics, ed 2. Lea & Febiger, Philadelphia, 1976.
28. Travell, JG and Rinzler SH: The myofascial genesis of pain. Postgrad Med 11:425–434, 1952.
29. Travell, JG and Simon, DG: Myofascial Pain and Dysfunction: The Trigger Point Manual. Williams & Wilkins, Baltimore, 1983, p 18.
30. Fischer, AA: Thermography and pain. Arch Phys Med Rehabil 62:542, 1981.
31. Travell, JG: Myofascial trigger points: Clinical view. In Bonica, JJ and Albe-Fessard, D (eds): Advances in Pain Research and Therapy, Vol 1. Raven Press, New York, 1976, pp 919–926.
32. Sola, AE and Kuitert, JH: Myofascial trigger point pain in the neck and shoulder girdle. Northwest Med 54:980–984, 1955.
33. Wilke, WS and Corbo, DD: Fibrositis/fibromyalgia: Causes and treatment. Compr Ther 15(1):28–34, 1989.
34. Cailliet, R: Abnormalities of the sitting postures of musicians. Medical Problems of Performing Artists 5(4):131–135, 1990.
35. Cailliet, R and Gross, L: The Rejuvenation Strategy. Doubleday, New York, 1987.
36. Cailliet, R: Shoulder Pain, ed 3. FA Davis, Philadelphia, 1991, pp 227–234.
37. Griffen, SJ and Trinder, J: Physical fitness, exercise and human sleep. Psychophysiology 15:447–450, 1978.
38. McCain, GA: Role of physical fitness training in the fibrositis/fibromyalgia syndrome. Am J Med 81:73–77, 1986.
39. Dworkin, RH and Gitlin, MJ: Clinical aspects of depression in chronic pain patients. Clin J Pain 7:79–94, 1991.

CHAPTER 8

Posttraumatic Headache

Modern life situations result in many head injuries and posttraumatic headaches. It has been estimated that 325,000 cases of mild head injuries occur annually in the United States, at a cost of over $1 billion for hospitalization.[1] Fully 42 percent of mild head injuries result from motor vehicular accidents; falls account for another 23 percent, and assaults 12 percent.[2] Falls occur mostly in the very young or the elderly. Ninety percent of trauma to the central nervous system results from head injury.

Although many head injuries are mild and cause no major functional impairment, they may present with subtle brain impairment termed *postconcussion syndrome*. Headache is a prominent symptom that often persists after the expected tissue swelling has subsided (30 to 50 percent for more than 2 months).[3] A headache that persists longer than 2 months is termed a *chronic posttraumatic headache*.

The severity of a posttraumatic headache cannot be related to the severity of the trauma using perimeters such as amnesia, coma, intracranial pressure elevation, or electroencephalographic changes.[4] Many severe posttraumatic headaches occur after relatively trivial injuries.[5]

A muscle tension type of headache may persist in these posttrauma cases. The sensory nerves located under the scalp may cause a neuralgia, with persistent pain and head tenderness. Migraine headaches have been claimed to result from head trauma.

The symptoms of a typical posttraumatic head injury syndrome are:

1. Vertigo
2. Tinnitus
3. Impaired memory
4. Reduced attention span
5. Easy distractibility

6. Deterioration of logical thinking
7. Insomnia
8. Apathy
9. Fatigability
10. Reduced motivation
11. Irritability
12. Mood swings
13. Anxiety, depression
14. Syncopal attacks

POSTTRAUMATIC STRESS SYNDROMES

The diagnosis of posttraumatic stress disorder (PTSD) was introduced into the American Psychiatric Association's official diagnostic manual in 1987.[6] Trauma is described as an event outside the range of normal human experience.

In the posttraumatic reaction—which may begin days, weeks, months, or even years after the trauma—there are three types of symptoms: First, the victim reexperiences the traumatic experience in the form of intrusive memories, nightmares, and vivid flashbacks during which he or she feels and acts as if the event were recurring. This recall may be inaccurate or distorted. Alternating with these memories is the occurrence of avoidance and emotional amnesia. The victim tries to avoid feelings, thoughts, discussion, and persons reminiscent of the event. Finally, there is hypersensitivity—irritability, edginess, nervousness, poor sleep patterns, and difficulty in concentrating.[7]

PTSD is usually accompanied by depression, often major, panic, grief, phobias, and even elements of chronic brain syndrome. Subtle intellectual defects may develop such as memory deficit and reduction of creativity. Intellectual, emotional, and physical fatigue may result from PTSD. Intellectual activity such as reading or writing may be initiated and discontinued shortly because of fatigue and even exertional headaches. These postconcussion syndrome patients apparently can only process small portions of information before experiencing fatigue and inattention.

Why certain posttrauma victims develop PTSD remains conjectural. Some psychologists postulate that an episode in adulthood exacerbates an unresolved childhood psychic trauma.[8] Patients suffering from PTSD after a single severe trauma have been reluctant to accept the concept of predisposition, especially in today's litigious society.

The significance of the trauma remains hard to relate specifically to the psychological aftermath. The failure to precisely remember the event has lead to this dilemma. Personality disorder predisposing to PTSD has also failed to be defined. Veterans of the Vietnam War have constituted much of current literature and are the focus of studies.[9] These studies have revealed a high degree of depression, anxiety, alcoholism, and drug abuse in family members or in victims pre trauma.

Patients with PTSD tend to retreat from or avoid exposure to any situation resembling the original trauma. This vigilance causes a state of detachment and isolation, and the individual becomes either hypersensitive or insensitive to their immediate environment.

Extreme stress causes significant changes in the chemistry of the brain such as alteration in neurotransmitters, especially catecholamines. Changes in catecholamine transmission result in less REM sleep, less stage 4 deep sleep, and more dreaming during non-REM sleep. This results in nightmares and nonrefreshing sleep.

The endogenous opiates are also affected in PTSD, causing an alteration in handling pain. This has been produced experimentally by stimulating the locus coeruleus, which sensitizes the neuroreceptors causing a psychological picture similiar to PTSD. This sensitivity may explain the susceptibility of PTSD to develop alcohol dependence.

PATHOMECHANICS OF HEAD TRAUMA

Initially all symptoms of head trauma sequelae were considered to be emotional, a result of hysteria and even malingering.[10,11] These opinions were held because of lack of documented pathological changes within the central nervous system thus implying that it "had to be emotional." The premorbid personality was indicated.[12] The advent of animal models and the clinical use of MRI studies revealed the presence of pathology.[13] Neck injuries associated with head trauma were also implicated.[14–16]

There are numerous microscopic brain changes that result from head trauma.[16] The physical properties of the skull and the contained brain determine the severity of the head injury. The skull cannot change in a closed head injury but the contained brain can become distorted, deformed, and traumatized within the skull. It is interesting that closed head injuries often cause greater residual impairment than a skull fracture; in the latter case the rigidity of the skull is changed, altering the hydrodynamics within the skull.

In acceleration-deceleration injuries the head moves upon the cervical spine.[17] The brain within the skull undergoes anterior-posterior and rotational shears and stresses. Contusions of the brain may occur from contact with the bony eminences of the internal skull. This brain motion has been documented in rhesus monkeys.[18] Wallerian degeneration of nerve fibers has been documented,[19] as well as small blood vessel injuries within the brain substance.[20] Some of the neurones injured apparently fail to recover

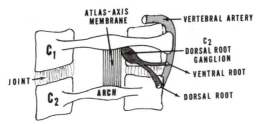

Figure 8–1. Greater superior occipital nerve emergence.

The C_2 dorsal ganglion lies under the obliquus inferior muscle (not shown) over the lateral atlantoaxial point. It is adherent upon the capsule with fascia. The C_2 nerve emerges lateral to the posterior atlas-axial membrane and does not penetrate it. It passes on laterally to divide into a dorsal and ventral root. (From Cailliet, R: Neck and Arm Pain, ed 3. FA Davis, Philadelphia, 1991, p 28, with permission.)

even after resolution of the edema and microscopic hemorrhage. There probably also occurs interruption of axonal connections.

Rebound of the brain—termed *contracoup*—also occurs, causing a double impact on the brain, with associated shear forces. Internal fluid imbalance may also result in a hydrocephalic change within the skull.[21,22]

The exact mechanism whereby headache results from brain injury remains conjectural. Vasoconstriction, edema, and autoregulation of the cerebrovascular tree have all been implicated, but the final decision has not been made. Trauma to the periductal gray region has been imputed.[23] Studies have also demonstrated that cerebral circulation is slowed for months to years after a head injury.[24] Other neurological abnormalities have been found following head trauma that invoke organic changes. These include abnormal brainstem–evoked potential,[25] impaired visual–evoked potentials,[26] as well as altered neurotransmitter function.[27]

Many head injuries also cause acceleration-deceleration injuries to the upper cervical spinal segement (occiput-atlas-axis).[17] The causation here is traumatic insult to the C-2 root as it emerges from lateral to the interosseous ligament (Fig. 8–1).

That headaches may stem from cervical injuries seems evident, but much remains unclear (see Chapter 6). Studies directed to the suboccipital region refer to the C-2 root as being the major sensory component of the greater occipital nerve (GON) have implicated entrapment within the involved neck muscles. The relationship of the GON to the contiguous muscles such as the semispinalis, the trapezius, and the inferior oblique muscles (which are injured in rear-end collisions) has been alluded to as significant.

The course of the greater occipital nerve and the nuchal muscles has recently been studied.[28] Autopsies show that the trapezius muscle was penetrated in 45 percent of the cases by the GON, whereas the semispinalis muscle was penetrated in 90 percent of cases dissected. The inferior oblique muscle was penetrated by the GON in only 7.5 percent of cases. There was microscopic evidence of nerve compression in 27 percent of cases. It appears that myogenic nerve entrapment of the greater occipital nerve with resultant headache following acceleration-deceleration injuries may be a valid conclusion. A recent study of muscular symptoms in patients with chronic headache revealed that "tightness" rather than soreness of the neck muscles was noted in chronic headache patients.[29]

An unexpected injury causes more damage than does the anticipated impact both to the brain as well as to the cervical spinal column. This possibly explains the lack of concussion in athletes.[17] It also explains the concept of Denny-Brown and Russell, who demonstrated in cats that less force was needed to produce concussion when the head was free as when it was fixed.[24]

CLINICAL EVALUATION OF THE HEAD TRAUMA PATIENT

The diagnosis depends upon a careful, thorough history as the objective findings may be minimal. Initially, a head trauma must be evaluated to elicit the major catastrophic types of head trauma that require urgent if not emergent care. These conditions include skull fracture, traumatic dissection of the extracranial internal carotid artery, intracranial epidural, subdural, and subarachnoid hemorrhage, rupture of an arteriovenous fistula, or acute hydrocephalus. Proper diagnostic studies can reveal these conditions after a careful history and neurological examination. These special studies consist of MRI, CT scan, spinal fluid studies, etc. (see Chapter 9).

In head trauma, victims' vital signs must be carefully evaluated and monitored. Hypoxia is noted in a large majority of patients who do not necessarily manifest respiratory difficulty.[30] Trauma enhances cerebral edema with intracranial pressure elevation. Cardiac arrhythmia further complicates the total picture, as does hypertensive response.[31] A basilar skull fracture should also be ruled out requiring evaluation of a Battle sign: discoloration behind the ears near the mastoid processes. Mobilization of the head and neck during the examination and special testing must be performed very carefully to avoid irreparable cervical cord injury.

The cranial nerves must be individually examined. Anosmia (loss of sense of smell) may result from damage by cribiform plate injury to cranial nerve I. Extraoccular motion and pupillary response must be evaluated. Injury to cranial nerve III may result in a dilated pupil and impaired upward-downward gaze. Diplopia may result from VIth nerve involvement. The trigeminal and facial nerve examination has been discussed in Chapter 4. Shoulder shrugging is a function of cranial nerve XI; the gag response tests nerves IX and X; tongue movement tests cranial nerve XII. Upper motor neurone tests for spasticity—monoplegia, paraplegia, or quadriplegia—must be elicited by examination of the deep tendon reflexes, Hoffmann and Babinski testings, etc.

Most patients with a closed head injury with or without headache have a negative neurological examination. The mental sequelae have been enumerated and include intellectual impairment, cognitive problems, and personality changes. These tests are numerous so a head trauma patient is best referred to a rehabilitation center or a neurosurgical service where all components of the team are available for an evaluation.[32]

The headache that presents after head trauma is often a headache that is generalized, bilateral, aching, and associated with scalp sensitivity over the involved portion of the head and with the many sequelae previously listed. Although a posttraumatic headache may be noted immediately, it must be remembered that the headache may be delayed.

DIAGNOSTIC STUDIES

Electroencephalographic studies are indicated if there is evidence of epileptic seizures, but these tests are currently being supplemented by cortical-evoked potential testing, brainstem-related potentials, and electronystagmographic testing.

MRI and CT scan are routinely evaluated when the head trauma has significant sequelae or symptomatology. CT scan is more universally available and less expensive, but MRI studies are considered more diagnostic and localizing. After the acute stage of the head injury subsides, an MRI proves more diagnostic. Contusions of the brain are visible on MRI studies.[33] MRI may reveal small subdural and epidural hemorrhages that may be missed on CT scan.[34] X-rays to the head and neck are needed if fracture or subluxation and dislocation are suspected. The literature regarding these tests is massive.[35]

The neuropsychological manifestations of head trauma are more specifically localized in coup-contracoup injuries and less discrete in acceleration-deceleration injuries.[34] Most cognitive and intellectual impairment incurred after head trauma disappears within 1 year after the trauma.

More recently a report of the organic factors involved in PTSD supported the findings of microscopic organic changes in this syndrome.[36] Unfortunately, objective findings have rarely been described as most closed head injuries do not undergo pathological autopsy studies. In the few cases that were studied there was noted a loss of nerve cells in the microglia and axons,[37] with neural fiber degeneration.[38,39]

There does not appear to be a relationship between periods of unconsciousness related to trauma and severity of the sequelae. Nor is severity a factor of litigation.[40]

**Table 8–1. PARTIAL CLASSIFICATION OF
POSTTRAUMATIC HEADACHE**

Traumatic neuralgias
    Trigeminal neuralgia
    Facial or oral trauma
    Fracture of facial bones

Extracranial trauma
    Contusion laceration hematoma
    Muscle contraction headache

Intracranial trauma
    Subdural, epidural, subarachnoid hematoma
    Arteriovenous fistula or rupture
    Hydrocephalus

Migraine, migraine variant, cluster headache

Neck injuries
    Acceleration-deceleration injuries
    Subluxations
    Fracture dislocations

MANAGEMENT OF POSTTRAUMATIC HEADACHE

It is mandatory that the more severe causes of posttraumatic headache, such as subdural and epidural hemorrhages and acute hydrocephalus, be identified to ensure immediate neurosurgical attention: decompression, vascular repair, shunting, or injection of anesthetic or steroidal solution. The suspicion of a severe aspect of head trauma initiates appropriate studies such as CT scan or MRI studies that lead to immediate intervention.

Superficial injuries such as contusion, scalp lacerations, hematomas, and galeal muscle may cause head pain, but they are readily discernable and respond rapidly to palliative local treatment.

Trauma to the head that persists may be one of the many chronic daily headaches that have been mentioned in Chapter 4. See also Table 8–1.

Management depends on the type of headache, as outlined in Chapter 4 and in Table 8–2.

Many of the complaints of the head-injured are subjective, prolonged, nonresponsive to numerous treatments, and unaccountable by objective diagnostic studies. This situation is unacceptable to the patients, the spouse, and the family. The patient's memory, attention span, sexual function, and ability to enjoy ordinary activities may be impaired, and depression may result from frustration. A sensible scientific explanation of the symptoms to the patient, spouse, family, lawyer, and insurance carrier tends to eliminate other aspects of anxiety, depression, anger, and noncompliance.[41–44]

Table 8–2. MANAGEMENT OF POSTTRAUMATIC HEADACHE

Surgical
    Decompression, repair, and local injection treatment
Medical
    Nonspecific
        Nonsteroidal anti-inflammatory medication
        Acetaminophen
        Tricyclic antidepressants
        Beta-adrenogenic blocking agents
        Monoamine oxidase inhibitor
        Avoidance of narcotics, tranquilizers, sedatives*
    Specific
        Migraine
            Ergotamine
            Calcium ion antagonist
        Cluster
            Oxygen inhalation
            Ergotamine
            Corticosteroid
            Lithium
            Metysergide
Physical modalities
    Traction: mechanical and/or manual
    Collar
    Exercise: ADL training
    Biofeedback
    Transcutaneous electrical nerve stimulation (TENS)
    Operant conditioning
Psychological intervention

*The use of narcotics is contraindicated in head injuries as it confuses the diagnostic procedures, gives false reassurance, and leads to addiction and dependence. Tranquilizers also add cognitive and intellectual aberrations, thus confusing the organic component.

The diagnosis of posttraumatic syndrome, because of paucity of objective organic findings, either on examination or by laboratory studies, remains a diagnosis of exclusion. Only if comprehensive neurocognitive studies are not performed adequately and appropriately interpreted does the diagnosis remain obscure—much to the detriment of our patients and their families.

REFERENCES

1. Report of the Panel on Strokes, Trauma, Regeneration and Neoplasms to the National Advisory Neurological and Communicative Disorders and Stroke Council. National Institutes of Health, Washington, DC, 1979.

2. Caveness, WF: Incidence of cranial cerebral trauma in the United States. Ann Neurol 1:507, 1977.

3. Brenner, CT, Friedman, AF, Merritt, HH, and Denny-Brown, D: Posttraumatic headache. Ann Neurosurg 1:379, 1944.

4. Friedman, AP and Merritt, HH: Relationship of intracranial pressure in the presence of blood in the cerebrospinal fluid to the occurrence of headache in patients with injuries to the head. J Nerv Ment Dis 102:1–7, 1945.

5. Miller, H: Accident neurosis. Br Med J 919–925, 992–993, 1961.

6. American Psychiatric Association: Diagnostic and Statistical Manual of Mental Disorders, ed 3 rev. American Psychiatric Association, Washington, DC, 1987.

7. Wolf, ME and Mosnaim, AD (eds): Post-Traumatic Stress Disorder: Etiology, Phenomenology and Treatment. American Psychiatric Press, Washington, DC, 1990.

8. Van der Kolk, BA: Psychological Trauma. American Psychiatric Press, Washington, DC, 1987.

9. Breslau, N and Davis, GC: Post-traumatic stress disorder: The stressor criterion. J Nerv Ment Dis 170:255–264, 1987.

10. Trimble, MR: Posttraumatic Neurosis. John Wiley & Sons, Chichester, 1981.

11. Page, H: Injuries of the Spine and Spinal Cord without Apparent Mechanical Lesions. J&H Churchill, London, 1985.

12. Lishman, WA: MR imaging of brain contusions. Psychol Med 3:304–318, 1973.

13. Hesselink, JR, Dowd, CF, Healy, ME et al: Am J Roentgenology 150:1133–1142, 1988.

14. Jacome, DE: Headache 26:515–516, 1986.

15. Khurana, RK and Nirankari, VS: Headache 26:183–188, 1986.

16. Bakay, L and Glasauer, FE: Head Injury. Little, Brown & Co, Boston, 1980.

17. Cailliet, R: Neck and Arm Pain, ed 3. FA Davis, Philadelphia, 1991, pp 81–123.

18. Pudenz, RH and Sheldon, CH: The lucite calvarium. A method for direct observation of the brain. J Neurosurg 3:487, 1946.

19. Strich, SJ: Diffuse degeneration of the cerebral white matter in severe dementia following head injury. J Neurol Neurosurg Psychiatry 19:163–185, 1956.

20. Peerless, SJ and Rewcastle, NB: Shear injuries of the brain. Can Med Assoc J 98:577–582, 1967.

21. Beyerl, B and Black, PM: Neurosurg 15:257–261, 1984.

22. Raskin, NH, Hosobuchi, Y, and Lamb, S: Headache 27:416–420, 1987.

23. Taylor, AR: The cerebral circulatory disturbance associated with the late effects of head injury. In Walker, AE, Caveness, WF and Critchley, M (eds): Late Effects of Head Injury. Charles C Thomas, Springfield, IL, 1969.

24. Denny-Brown, D and Russell, WR: Experimental cerebral concussion. Brain 64:93, 1941.

25. Noseworthy, JH, Miller J, Murray, TJ, and Regan, D: Auditory brain stem evoked responses in postconcussion syndrome. Arch Neurol 38:275–278, 1981.

26. Ommaya, AK and Gennarelli, TA: Cerebral concussion and traumatic unconsciousness. Brain 97:633–754, 1970.

27. Van Woerkom, TCAM, Teelken, AW, and Minderhond, JM: Difference in neurotransmitter metabolism in fronto-temporal lobe contusion and diffuse cerebral contusion. Lancet 1:812–813, 1977.

28. Bovim, G, Bonamico, L, Torbjorn, AF, Lindboe, CF, Stolt-Nielson, A, and Sjaastad, O: Topographic variations in the peripheral course of the greater occipital nerve: Autopsy study with clinical correlations. Spine 16(4):475–478, 1991.

29. Lebbink, J, Spierings, ELH, and Messinger, HB: A questionnaire survey of muscular symptoms in chronic headache: An age- and sex-controlled study. Clin J Pain 7:95–101, 1991.

30. Katsurada, K, Yamada, R, and Sugimoto, T: Respiratory insufficiency in patients with severe head injuries. Surgery 73:191–219, 1973.

31. Vander Ark, GD: Comments on respiratory problems associated with head trauma. Surg Neurol 3:305–308, 1975.
32. Jennett, B and Teasdale, G: Management of Head Injuries. FA Davis, Philadelphia, 1981.
33. Hyman, RA and Gorey, MT: Radiol Clin North Am 26:471–503, 1988.
34. Zimmerman, RD, Snow, RB, Gandy, SE, et al: Radiology 153:344, 1984.
35. Elkind, AH: Headache and Facial Pain. Raven Press, New York, 1990, pp 273–299.
36. Lezak, MD: Neuropsychological Assessment, ed 2. Oxford University Press, New York, 1983.
37. Speed, WG: Closed head injury sequelae: Changing concepts. Headache 29:643–647, 1989.
38. Strich, SJ: The pathology of brain damage due to blunt head injury. In Walker, AE, Caveness, WF, and Critchley, S (eds): Late Effects of Head Injury. Charles C Thomas, Springfield, IL, 1969, pp 501–526.
39. Oppenheimer, DR: Microscopic lesions in the brain following head injury. J Neurol Neurosurg Psychiatry 31:299, 1968.
40. Leininger, BE: Neuropsychological deficits in symptomatic minor head injury patients after concussion and mild concussion. J Neurol Neurosurg Psychiatry 53:293–296, 1990.
41. Denker, PG: The post-concussion syndrome: Prognosis and evaluation of organic factors. NY State J Med 271:379–384, 1943.
42. Kelly, R and Smith, BN: Post-traumatic syndrome: Another myth discredited. J R Soc Med 74:275–277, 1981.
43. Balla, J and Moraitis, S: Knight in armor: A follow-up study of injuries after legal settlement. Med J Aust 2:355–361, 1970.
44. Stuss, DT, et al: Subtle neuropsychological deficits in patients with good recovery after closed head injury. Neurosurgery 17:41–47, 1985.

CHAPTER 9

Neurosurgical Aspects of Headache

Because of the many nociceptor sites of pain within the head, it is mandatory that any cause demanding neurosurgical evaluation and intervention be immediately recognized. Among these nociceptor sites are the pericranium, periosteum of the skull, upper cervical spine, blood vessels of the scalp, external auditory canal, tympanic membrane, dura within the skull (Fig. 9–1), the blood vessels of the dura, falx cerebri, tentorium, and many of the venous sinuses. Any of these can be involved in head trauma or tumor growths that may have neurosurgical impact.

Some structures that can be traumatically involved are not pain-sensitive, so their involvement can be identified only by impairment, disability, and incidental findings when performing a neurological examination. They may be suggested by x-rays, MRI, and CT scans. These insensitive structures are the brain parenchyma, ependyma, choroid plexus, pia mater, arachnoid matter, and the bony skull itself. The periosteum of the skull, however, is pain-sensitive.

The intracranial blood vessels at the base of the brain are well innervated by sympathetic nerve fibers which transmit pain sensation. They ascend into the cranial cavity within the internal carotid artery wall. Many of the internal cranial cavity contents above the tentorium are supplied by the trigeminal nerve. Below the tentorium they are supplied by the glossopharyngeal and vagus nerves.

The sensation of pain is delineated by the tentorium. Pain emanating from below the tentorium is felt in the occipital area and from above the tentorium in the frontal, parietal, and temporal areas. Pain arising from the sympathetic innervation of the internal carotid artery is usually felt in the region of and behind the eye.

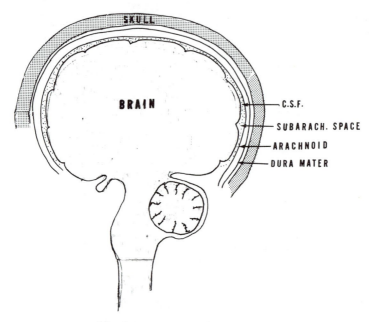

Figure 9–1. Covering of the brain.

Under the skull is the dura mater: a tough fibrous membrane. Next is the lining of the brain, the pia arachnoid, which is thin and transparent. Beneath the arachnoid and between it and the brain is the spinal fluid.

The role of the innervation of blood vessels causing pain from the internal cranial substances has been clarified.[1] These vessels are especially the proximal part of the cerebral and dural arteries, the large veins, the venous sinuses, and the dural arteries.

The internal and external carotid arteries are supplied from sympathetic fibers emanating from the carotid plexus, which receives branches from C-8, T-1, and T-2. The vagus and upper thoracic spinal nerves transmit fibers to the carotid nerve plexus, and the carotid artery may receive branches from the IIId, IVth, and VIth cranial nerves. The scalp is amply supplied by branches of the external carotid artery, which experiences pain when distended or stretched.

A mass lesion within the cranium often causes pain by displacing a major blood vessel or by increasing intracranial pressure and stretching the dura, a pain-sensitive structure. Obstruction of the cerebral spinal fluid resulting in hydrocephalus causes pain in the same manner. Direct pressure from tumor against the trigeminal or vagus nerves can also cause head pain.

Increased intracranial pressure causes headache. The intracranial pressure is well regulated as the contents of the skull—the brain, the cerebrospinal fluid (Fig. 9–2), the blood vessels, the meninges, and the blood vessels—are maintained in balance. Any change in the volume of any of the

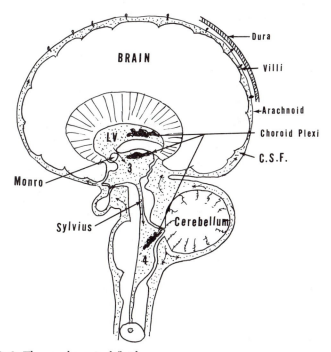

Figure 9–2. The cerebrospinal fluid.

The source of the cerebrospinal fluid (C.S.F.) is believed to be the choroid plexi with 95% formed in the two lateral ventricles (LV) which connect by the interventricular foramen of Monro. From there it circulates through the interventricular foramen into the third ventricle (3) then into the fourth ventricle (4) via the aqueduct of Sylvius. From the fourth ventricle it circulates into the subarachnoid spaces surrounding the brain.

The fluid is finally absorbed by the subarachnoid villi which project into the dural venous sinuses.

components happens at the expense of the other components within the fixed space of the rigid skull. Headache is often the first sign of increased intracranial pressure and is especially noted in rapidly growing tumors which preclude adjustment of the pressure variants.[2]

ACUTE INTRACRANIAL HEMORRHAGE

Intracranial hemorrhage, usually the result of trauma, is usually severe, disabling, and even life-threatening. Hemorrhage may occur in the subarachnoid, intracranial, epidural, or subdural regions. Fortunately, many of these are amenable to surgical correction without severe residual damage. Early recognition is therefore paramount to ensure proper treatment.

Subarachnoid Hemorrhage

Spontaneous subarachnoid hemorrhage produces an excruciating explosive headache with gradual coma, stiff neck (not necessarily noted immediately), and variable neurological findings. A cough headache may also indicate elevated intracranial pressure. Subarachnoid hemorrhage may result from trauma, but there are nontraumatic causes as well.

In 75 percent of subarachnoid hemorrhage of nontraumatic etiology, rupture of an aneurysm is the cause.[3] A rupture of an arteriovenous malformation may also be the etiology. Headache results from the rush, under pressure, of blood into the subarachnoid space. This upsets the balance within the cranial cavity. An obstructive hydrocephalus results, as does irritation of the meninges and the cranial nerves. A stiff neck often occurs and coma is not unusual. The blood within the space breaks down into catecholamines, serotonin, phospholipids, and prostaglandin, which are nociceptors and vasoconstrictors. The resultant vasoconstriction (vasospasm) also enhances headache.

The offending structures (aneurysm or malformation) may rerupture within a period of time after the initial rupture, resulting in a recurrent severe headache. Prior to rupture the offending vessels may dilate, producing a premonitory headache. This headache may be felt in the distribution of the trigeminal nerve or by pressure upon other nerves such as the third cranial nerve and its sequelae (pupilary changes). Headache may also result from the violation of the tentorium. When an expanding aneurysm is suspected, an angiogram should be performed to allow surgical intervention before rupture.

As there are numerous sources of the subarachnoid hemorrhage, its identification begins with a noncontrast CT scan. The basal cisterns will appear filled with blood and the site of aneurysmal rupture can also be identified. A CT scan must be done early as it becomes less specifically diagnostic within days when the blood elements break down and the density of the blood decreases.

A lumbar puncture should always be performed, as it is often diagnostic of the presence of blood. The bloody spinal fluid remains for several days so it need not be an emergent procedure although immediate recognition of a bloody spinal fluid alerts the examiner to the need for other tests.[4] An aneurysm must be ruled out even with a negative lumbar puncture when there is an abrupt severe explosive headache. CT or MRI studies are indicated even with a normal spinal fluid.

Intracranial Hemorrhage

Intracranial hemorrhage should be suspected when there is severe headache followed by coma of a variable degree and gradual signs of hemiplegia:

at first flaccid then spastic.[5] There is a high correlation between intracranial hemorrhage, aging, and preexisting hypertension or diabetes. A CT scan may be diagnostic. Treatment is of the sequelae by means of physical, occupational, and speech therapy.[6]

The often experienced transient ischemic attack (TIA) with no residual sequelae is not usually accompanied by headache, although some authors claim there is headache in 25 percent of cases.[7]

Epidural Hematoma

An epidural hematoma is an accumulation of blood between the outer layer of the dura and the inner table of the skull. This condition usually occurs as the result of head trauma at the temporal area, where the bone is thin and the underlying meningeal artery is vulnerable.

The dura is not firmly attached to the inner table of the skull in young people, and a hematoma can expand easily in this space with subsequent traction and tearing of the associated blood vessels. This results in increasing progressive hemorrhage from the tearing of the blood vessels.

The dura is a well-innervated pain-sensitive tissue. The hemorrhage stretches and irritates the dura, resulting in headache and coma. Because hemorrhage is arterial it progresses rapidly with ominous results within 20 to 30 minutes. The diagnosis relies upon a history of trauma, acute excruciating explosive headache, progressive loss of consciousness, an ipsilateral dilated pupil, and contralateral hemiparesis. A CT scan confirming the diagnosis mandates immediate surgical intervention: a burr hole must be drilled; there must be an adequate airway and respiratory assistance; and Mannitol is administered to decrease associated cerebral edema. Evacuation of the hematoma may be life-saving.

Subdural Hematoma

When hemorrhage occurs between the dura and the underlying pia arachnoid membrane lining the brain, the condition is termed *subdural hematoma*. This condition usually occurs within hours of a head trauma resulting in laceration of the brain in the region of the pia-arachnoid membrane. In many patients the damage is the residual of the brain injury rather than the sequential subdural hematoma. As many patients so afflicted become comatose, they cannot complain of pain, and thus the diagnosis may be delayed.

Because the elderly have "brittle" blood vessels and some degree of cortical atrophy, the hematoma may be insidious and follow a trivial injury. The hemorrage is usually slow venous oozing in the subdural space. Initially, internal balance is maintained and headache is a gradually increasing dull ache rather than severe and explosive. The symptoms are a gradual hemiparesis, speech difficulty, and commensurate neurological deficit. Insidious personality and mental changes may arouse suspicion.

POSTCONCUSSION HEADACHE

This condition has been discussed in the preceding chapter and will be noted here only for its consideration as a neurosurgical condition. Most are "closed head" injuries that require medical and not surgical attention.

BRAIN TUMORS CAUSING HEADACHE

Malignant glioma is a common brain tumor frequently causing headache, whereas a meningioma is a slower-growing tumor that may not cause headache. Cerebellopontine-angle tumors usually do not cause headaches until they reach a size that obstructs cerebrospinal fluid (CSF), resulting in a hydrocephalus.

A chronic, dull, aching headache together with vomiting and papilledema indicate increased intracranial pressure. The location of the headache is characteristic. A tumor within the posterior fossa is felt in the occipital area and upper neck. Supratentorial tumors cause a headache felt in the vertex temporal area or frontal region. Coughing or straining, which acutely increases CSF pressure, aggravates the headache.

The numerous types of tumor are beyond the scope of this text but are well documented in the literature, where the specific site, significance, rate of growth, diagnostic tests, and treatment are enumerated.[8]

PSEUDOTUMOR CEREBRI

Benign intracranial hypertension can present a confusing diagnostic picture by presenting a clinical picture of tumor with no tumor present. This condition is termed *pseudotumor cerebri* and is caused by an elevation of CSF with resultant papilledema. There may be significant headache and blurred vision.[9] Pseudotumor cerebri usually occurs in women of childbearing age.

There are numerous etiologies of pseudotumor cerebri, such as dural venous thrombosis, intracranial venous occlusion, adrenal insufficiency, hypoparathyroidism, and even prolonged corticosteroid medication. The findings suggestive of increased cerebrospinal pressure without tumor may be substantiated by MRI or CT studies. These studies fail to reveal displacement of the ventricular system but may demonstrate the absence of blood flow within the sinuses. The lumbar puncture testing will reveal elevated pressure with a clear cell-free fluid and normal protein.

Pseudotumor may occur as a complication of a chronic ear infection. The benign condition is usually self-limiting. If blindness appears imminent, surgical intervention by shunting is warranted.[10]

HEADACHE FROM DIMINISHED SPINAL FLUID PRESSURE

A lowering of spinal fluid pressure may cause headache. The lowering of CSF pressure is frequently noted after removal of CSF fluid in a spinal tap preoperatively, diagnostically, or therapeutically (such as in the treatment of hydrocephalus). It can be noted after the performance of a contrast study (a myelogram).

The headache, often severe, is brought on by sitting or standing and is relieved by lying horizontally. The headache is apparently caused by traction upon the dura and upper cervical nerves and is felt in the frontal area, the occiput, and the upper neck. A stiffness in the neck resembling meningitis may result.

Bed rest with forced fluid intake is usually therapeutic. Treatment by blood patch has been recommended: at the site of the lumbar puncture, epidural injection of several cc's of the patient's blood allegedly clots and closes the leak of CFS. More recently the benefit from a blood patch is being attributed to the increased pressure against the involved dura rather than from the clotting. Increased cerebrospinal pressure is accomplished by intravenous infusion of 500 cc of sterile fluid or an epidural infusion of a similiar amount of sterile fluid.

HEADACHE FROM CRANIAL INFECTION

Osteomyelitis of the skull can cause headache. This is usually secondary to infection of adjacent sinuses or is a blood-borne osteomyelitis. An epidural abscess may also occur as a complication of a sinus infection.

HEADACHE FROM CERVICAL SPINE TRAUMA

The relationship of headache with cervical spine pathology has been discussed in Chapter 5. The conditions requiring neurosurgical intervention are subluxation, dislocation, and fracture of cervical vertebral components with subsequent spinal cord compression.

OCCIPITAL NEURALGIA

This condition, also previously described, may require neurosurgical intervention as indicated by the severity and neurological impairment and disability. Therapeutic injections of an anesthetic agent and/or steroid may be administered by an anesthesiologist, a physiatrist, an orthopedist, or a well-trained general practitioner. Only when severity and failure to respond to treatment are imminent should a neurosurgeon's services be required.

REFERENCES

1. Ray, BS and Wolff, HG: Experimental studies on headache. Pain-sensitive structures of the head and their significance in headache. Arch Surg 41:813, 1940.
2. Kunkle, EC, Ray, BS, and Wolff, HG: Experimental studies on headache. Arch Neurol Psychiatry 49:323, 1943.
3. Sahs, AL: Subarachnoid hemorrhage. In Harrison, MJG and Dyken, ML (eds): Cerebral Vascular Disease. Butterworth, London, 1983, p 354.
4. Kassell, NF and Drake, CG: Timing of aneurysm surgery. Neurosurgery 10:514–519, 1982.
5. Cailliet, R: The Shoulder in Hemiplegia. FA Davis, Philadelphia, 1980.
6. Davies, PM: Steps to Follow. Springer-Verlag, New York, 1985.
7. Edmeads, J: The headache of ischemic cerebro-vascular disease. Headache 19:345–349, 1979.
8. Jennett, B and Teasdale, G: Management of Head Injuries. FA Davis, Philadelphia, 1981.
9. Rush, JA: Mayo Clin Proc 55:541–546, 1980.
10. Davies, G and Zilkha, KJ: Trans Ophthalmol Soc UK 99:427–429, 1976.

CHAPTER 10

Temporomandibular Joint Pain

Of the numerous face pains presenting to the clinician the complaint of temporomandibular joint (TMJ) arthralgia is increasingly frequent. The International Association for the Study of Headache has included this entity in the classification of atypical odonyalgia (see Table 10–1).[1]

The subdivisions of this classification relate principally to deviations of the disc wherein the disc deviates in its soft tissue form, including perforation, elongation, and narrowing associated with or without pain. Where displacement is noted, the condition is then classified according to whether the disc displacement reduces and whether there is pain and/or crepitation ("clicking") in the act of opening and closing the mouth.

The disc requires definition in structure and function. It is soft and pliable and undergoes physiological deformation (Fig. 10–1). The temporomandibular joint (TMJ) is essentially a universal joint operational about an incongruous joint structure with a shifting axis of rotation. Congruity has been described as the articular situation where the opposing surfaces have a different degree of arc.[2–4] In the TMJ the surface of the condyle is ovoid and the surface of the opposing joint is sellar (Fig. 10–2). Movement thus occurs as a gliding motion (Fig. 10–3) rather than as an arc rotation (Fig. 10–4).

The jaw opens, protrudes, retracts, laterally rotates, and undergoes a degree of circumduction as in a chewing manner. The temporomandibular joint is a diarthrodal synovial joint. These motions are permitted, directed, and limited by the articular surfaces, the texture of the meniscus, the ligaments, the capsular tissues, and the numerous muscles that operate the joint. It is a complex joint. In opening the mouth the first 25° are through rotation (ginglymal); the condyles then translate upon the glenoid fossa cartilage (arthrodial).

The degree that the mouth opens needs to be objectively measured. A

Table 10–1. TEMPOROMANDIBULAR DISORDERS

Deviation in form
Disc displacement with reduction
Disc displacement without reduction
Inflammation
Hypermobility
Osteoarthritis
Osteoarthropathy
Polyarthritides and connective tissue disorders
    Rheumatoid arthritis
    Psoriatic arthritis
    Ankylosing arthritis
    Systemic lupus erythematosus
    Scleroderma
Fibrous ankylosis
Bony ankylosis
Dislocation

simple instrument has been proposed to measure this opening (Fig. 10–5). It is inserted between the teeth in the midline. The degree of opening can be seen and recorded. The same instrument can also objectively measure the extent the jaw can be protruded.

There are numerous muscles that operate the jaw, and it is in these muscles that many of the complaints of facial pain originate. These are classified as muscle disorders.[1]

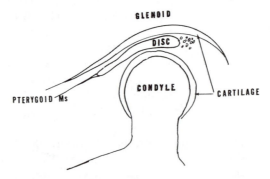

Figure 10–1. Temporomandibular joint.

The concavity of the glenoid fossa differs from the convexity of the mandibular condyle forming an incongruous joint. Both are covered with cartilage which physiologically deforms during motion. The disc is fibrocartilage in structure and is held and elongated by the pterygoid muscle.

Behind the disc are numerous blood vessels, lymphatics, and connective tissue fibers (shown by the dotted area).

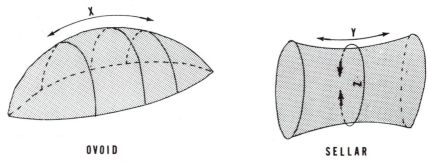

OVOID   **SELLAR**

Figure 10–2. Joint surfaces.

There are two basic joint surfaces: ovoid and sellar. The ovoid is uniformly convex (X) at each point along the surface. The sellar surface is convex (Z) in one plane and concave (Y) in the perpendicular plane. (From Cailliet, R: Shoulder Pain, ed 3. FA Davis, Philadelphia, 1991, p 5, with permission.)

    Myositis
    Myofascial pain
    Splinting/trismus
    Contracture
    Hypertrophy

Myositis is relatively infrequent, whereas myofascial pain is more frequently described and diagnosed.[5] This condition has been described in detail in Chapter 8, but the highlights related to TMJ syndrome can be enumerated. There are associated trigger areas in the muscle as well as deep tenderness with typical patterns of referral. The pain and tenderness is

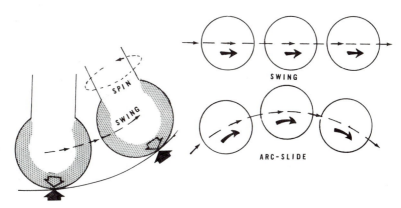

Figure 10–3. Joint motion.

Slide of a joint moving in one plane is termed *swing*. In this motion there is no rotation or spin. If there is simultaneous spin, the motion is termed *arc-slide*. (From Cailliet, R: Shoulder Pain, ed 3. FA Davis, Philadelphia, 1991, p 7, with permission.)

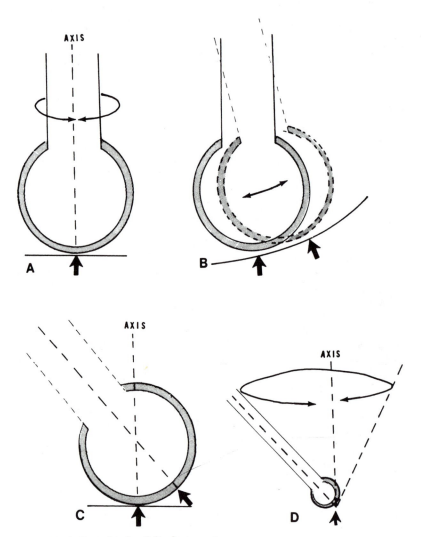

Figure 10–4. Basic kinds of displacement.
(A) True spin about an axis. (B) Arc slide called "swing" when there is no concurrent rotation or spin. (C) Spin about the axis of rotation. (D) Spin is rotation about an axis perpendicular to fixed surface. (Adapted from Licht, S (ed): Arthritis and Physical Medicine. Williams & Wilkins, Baltimore, 1969.)

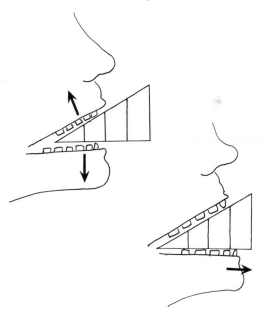

Figure 10–5. Plastic instrument to objectively measure opening and protrusion of the jaw.

A plastic firm card measures in inches the opening and protrusion of the jaw for clinical recording.

typically reduced by local muscle vasocoolant spray, injection, and gentle stretching.

Pain in the masticatory muscles can coexist with pain in cervical muscles as well as from the temporomandibular joint. These are specifically related but pose a differential diagnostic challenge as regard to their management. The term *TMJ syndrome* should probably be abandoned as it implies a common cause of this painful syndrome. This fact is rarely noted as many patients have pain and dysfunction without organic joint disease or articular malfunction and the opposite also can exist. A better term than TMJ syndrome would probably be *myofascial pain dysfunctional syndrome of the temporomandibular articulation.*

The syndrome only partially belongs in the domain of dentistry. The incidence of this syndrome is more common among females ages 30 to 60: 4:1 in myogenic and 9.5:1 in internal derangement.[6]

There appears to be a high incidence of joint hypermobility in patients who present with internal derangement.[7] Patients who have a preponderance of articular symptoms rather than muscular painful dysfunction present with clicking, crepitation, and bruxism. These patients also usually ultimately display changes on MRI studies, but as will be developed in discussing the concepts of the mechanisms of malfunction, the neuromuscular dysfunction precedes, in fact initiates and aggravates, the ultimate structural articular pathology.

Masticatory fibromyalgia is considered to be of muscular etiology if the symptomatology is bilateral, whereas if the symptoms and findings are initially unilateral, the condition is considered to be of articular etiology. The

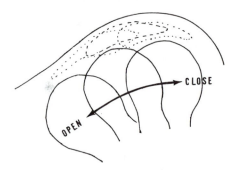

Figure 10–6. Deformation of the disc in jaw opening and closing.

The disc deforms rather than moves with the condyle as the jaw opens and closes. The drawing shows movement but the disc essentially deforms being held between the glenoid fossa and the moving condyle.

The cartilage of the condyle (not shown in this drawing) also deforms during movement.

masticatory type is also usually related to function (during chewing), and there are tender points noted within the masticatory muscles with a limited range of motion of the jaw. Crepitation is usually absent in this situation.

Dental abnormality may result and/or coexist. Whether these dental abnormalities are primary or secondary remains unanswered. This question implies that muscular dysfunction and asymmetry can ultimately cause organic dental alignment, whereas the original TMJ concept was that deviations of occlusion preceded and initiated ultimate temporomandibular disorder including the muscle disorder.

When a dental malocclusion is present, splints have been in vogue and effective. These orthodontics attempt to achieve the ideal vertical facial height, correct dental occlusion, and regain central position of the mandibular condyles within the glenoid fossae. Attempts at realignment have been disappointing, as the orthosis cannot accomplish all the requirements of proper occlusion, which include vertical overlap, cross-bite relationship, molar contact, and balance of the musculature.[8]

There are proprioceptor factors in mastication and balance of the "bite" present in the ligaments, joints, and capsules, and even in the spindle system of the masticatory muscles. These proprioceptor feedbacks are considered significantly involved in the pathology and therefore pertinent in reeducation of the patient with symptomatic masticatory dysfunction.[9]

The disc and the articular cartilages play a predominant role in normal joint motion and also in painful dysfunction. The cartilage of the glenoid fossa and that covering the condylar surface are fibrocartilagenous, unlike the condylar surfaces and menisci of other synovial joints. These articular tissues deform physiologically in all joint motions and especially so in the temporomandibular joint: flexion, extension, protrusion, retraction, lateral motion, and circumduction motion.

Contrary to the knee joint (Fig. 10–6), where the meniscus moves with the femur in rotation and with the tibia in flexion-extension,[10] the disc of the TMJ deforms (Fig. 10–7) during these motions and reforms after termination of motion. The undersurface of the disc is tightly attached to the

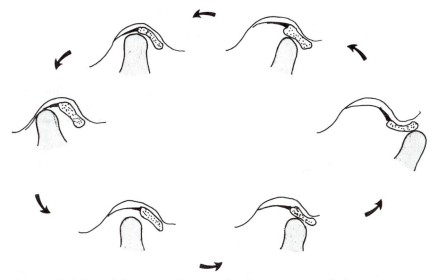

Figure 10–7. Disc deformation during cycle of jaw opening and closing.

As the jaw opens and closes, the disc deforms to accommodate the opening between the condyle and the glenoid fossa. The disc is held anteriorly by a filament to the pterygoid muscle (*dark line*) emanating from the anterior margin of the disc. Throughout the cycle of the jaw, the condyle moves anteriorly and posteriorly within the glenoid fossa.

condyle, and essentially both function as a unit. Only when the disc does not undergo adequate deformation and reformation during active motion does the joint "lock."

The disc (meniscus) is biconcave with a thick anterior band (pes), a thin middle zone (pars gracilis), and a thick posterior band (pars posterior) (see Fig. 10–1). Anteriorly, it is attached to the capsule and some fibers of the lateral pterygoid muscle. Medially and laterally, the disc attaches firmly to the joint capsule. Posteriorly, there is a fibrovascular zone (Fig. 10–1), which contains veins, elastic fibers, and dense connective tissue. This posterior zone is richly supplied by nerve endings of the auriculotemporal nerve, with additional contribution from the masseter and deep posterior temporal nerve branches of the third (mandibular) division of the trigeminal nerve.

In faulty mechanical action the disc may tear from the underlying condyle. Its fibrous attachments tear. The lateral pterygoid thus is able to dislocate the disc anteriorly.

The musculature that moves the mandible and the discs are as follows: The lateral pterygoids are the major abductors (opening) of the lower jaw (Fig. 10–8). The digastric muscles also abduct (open) the jaw (Fig. 10–9). The temporalis muscle (Fig. 10–10), the masseter muscle (Fig. 10–11), and the medial pterygoid muscles adduct (close) the mandible.

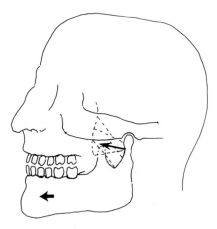

Figure 10–8. Lateral (external) pterygoid muscle.

The two divisions of the lateral pterygoid muscle lie deep to the zygomatic arch. The muscle originates from the infratemporal crest and the great wing of the sphenoid bone. It attaches to the neck of the condyle and the posterior superior aspect of the ramus of the mandible.

Its action is principally protrusion of the mandible, some lateral motion of the mandible, and has been found to be mildly active during opening of the jaw.

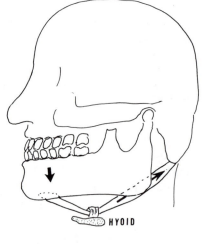

Figure 10–9. Digastric muscle.

The digastric muscle originates (posteriorly) from the mastoid process, passes through a fibrous loop attached to the hyoid bone, and then inserts to the midline of the undersurface of the mandible.

Its action is to open the jaw and influence some lateral opening.

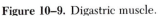

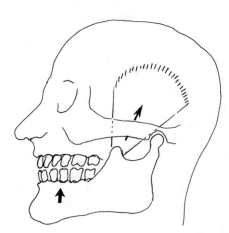

Figure 10–10. Temporalis muscle.

This muscle originates from the bone of the temporal fossa superior to the zygomatic arch. It attaches to the coronoid process of the mandible. Its action is elevation of the mandible and closes the mouth. In clenching the jaw tightly all fibers of the temporalis muscle contract.

In lateral jaw movements there is unilateral action with contralateral side relaxation. In opening the mouth the temporalis muscle relaxes appropriately.

Figure 10–11. Masseter muscle.

This muscle termed the Trismus Muscle is in two layers. Both layers originate from the zygomatic arch and insert to the external surface of the mandible at its angle, and the inferior half of the ramus. The deep layer attaches to the superior half of the ramus (*dotted lines*).

The action of the masseter muscle is elevation of the mandible closing the jaw. The deep fibers, by their angle, tend to slightly retrude the mandible.

The masseter must relax in the opening of the jaw. This muscle acts in conjunction with the temporalis but is stronger in bite force.

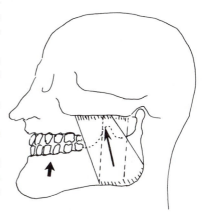

Normal function of the temporomandibular joint requires

- normal opening because of adequate dental occlusion, together with
    - normal shape and length of the teeth and
    - normal articular muscular action. The latter also depends upon
        - correct appropriate neuromuscular coordination, which is in turn achieved by
        - proprioceptive feedback from mechanoreceptors in the ligaments and the spindle system in the musculature. Pathology occurs when there is a breakdown of any or all of these areas:
        - appropriate, mechanical, ligamentous, limitation preventing hypermobility

Bruxism, an audible and occasionally painful condition, is the "grinding" of the teeth during sleep. The level of discomfort upon awakening and during daytime hours depends on its severity, duration, and frequency. The cause of bruxism remains unclear and is considered to be a sleep disturbance which fits into the definition of myofascial pain (see Chapter 7).[10] Bruxism is most destructive when it occurs during REM sleep. Bruxism occurring during stage II sleep apparently does not cause destructive dental or mandibular changes. Treating the sleep disorder is thus valid to prevent degenerative changes to the teeth and TMJ structures.[11]

Occlusal discrepancies are not considered pertinent to explain bruxism,[12] but splint therapy to correct malocclusion combined with sleep correction appears to be the most favorable approach.[13] It is of interest that bruxism recurs within a period of 2 weeks when these modalities are discontinued, suggesting that a complete holistic program is indicated rather than merely splinting and prescribing sleep medication.

CLINICAL MANIFESTATIONS OF
TEMPOROMANDIBULAR ARTHRALGIA

The clinical picture of TMJ arthralgia varies according to the causation, the etiology, the tissues involved, the symptomatology, and the diagnostic procedures invoked. Once the correct pathomechanical etiology and the involved tissue sites are ascertained, appropriate treatment follows.[14]

Possibly the most common type of temporomandibular arthralgia is a sequence of myofascial temporomandibular dysfunction. Pain that results from this disorder occurs mostly, at least in the initial stages, in the mastication muscles, especially the temporalis and masseter, which are undergoing sustained contraction from numerous causes. The sustained muscle contraction also initiates trigger points with localized muscular tenderness and even referred pain.

The sustained muscle contraction is itself painful (tension myositis). This was initially termed Costen's syndrome.[15] The symptoms were described as pain tenderness and joint dysfunction. Numerous concepts were entertained and numerous specialties became involved: dental, medical, rheumatological, psychological, radiological, and oral surgical. The constellation of symptoms lead to the more recent diagnosis of TMPDS: temporomandibular pain and dysfunction syndrome, which, interestingly, does not directly relate to anatomical structural change and symptomatology.

The symptoms are a dull, aching sensation of gradual increasing duration in the region of the temporomandibular joint. At times pain is severe. It is felt anterior to the ear and radiates into the lateral temporal face and head region. Pain is aggravated by teeth clenching, biting, and chewing. The masticatory muscles become tender. There gradually results limited jaw opening, which may be accompanied by audible and palpable clicking or crepitation of the temporomandibular joint. Nocturnal and even diurnal bruxism is frequently noted.[16] Level IV sleep disturbances are frequent without restorative benefit. The incidence of temporomandibular arthralgia and myalgia is more frequent in females, usually in early adulthood.

At first there may be no precise dental abnormalities but as time ensues some secondary changes may be noted. Dental malocculsion may have previously existed and been asymptomatic but now become symptomatic and are considered to be the primary basis for TMJ. In time, changes in the cartilage of the condyles and/or glenoid fossae can result and enhance the basis of pain and joint limitation.

Faulty neuromuscular function may lead to meniscal (disc) disturbance with internal derangement.[17,18] Pain aggravates the neurological dysfunction by adding sustained muscular contraction as related to pain.[19] Stressful life situations may coexist and may have actually precipitated the entire syndrome. In an attempt to find a psychological predisposition for TMPDS patients recent studies have not found most patients significantly different from non-TMPDS patients when evaluated by psychological inventories.[20] Psychological improvement in patients with a profile of disturbance resulted from the amelioration of the condition rather than from psychological intervention.[21]

DIFFERENTIAL DIAGNOSIS OF TMJ PAIN

Evaluation of patients with TMJ pain should include a thorough history, a physical examination, and a radiological examination. The physical examination should determine:

1. Range of motion of the mandible

    • Sagittal (vertical) opening
    • Horizontal plane (protrusion, retraction, and lateral)
    • Objective measurement
    • Deviation and deflection of the mandible

2. Joint noises during motion (crepitation, clicking)
3. Pain location (subjective and by examination)
4. Palpation of muscles, joints, and ligaments

The problems causing the temporomandibular arthralgia can be divided into intracapsular and/or extracapsular. Intracapsular TMJ arthralgia includes closed lock, degenerative articular changes, subluxation, and displaced disc causing clicking. The latter is evaluated by palpation, mandibular deviation, range of motion, and radiological confirmation. Extracapsular TMJ arthralgia includes dysfunction of the masseter, temporal, medial pterygoid, and lateral pterygoid muscles.

Injury to the mandible with damage to the meniscus is a dreaded sequela of the initial temporomandibular arthralgia. There are numerous forms of pathology of the disc, including perforation, thinning, and thickening of the disc; changes that result in folded, vascularized, dislocated, or ankylosed disc; and ridges on the disc. There may be cartilaginous and bone changes of the temporomandibular joint as well as capsular changes.

Injury that merely disrupts the attachment of the meniscus to the condyle allows the pterygoid muscle to dislocate the meniscus in an anteromedial direction. When the patient attempts to open the mouth, the condyle encroaches upon the disc as it moves forward and causes a clicking sound, often with pain. If there has been a reduction of the prolapsed disc, complete forward motion of the condyle will recur and the jaw will open. If the entrapped disc has not been reduced, movement will remain limited, and the joint locked. Disc dislocations may be divided into nonpainful and painful types. In a painful locked dislocation, the type is termed as reducible or nonreducible.

When there have been repeated dislocations with or without reduction, the cartilage of the glenoid and the condyle undergo damage and degeneration with resultant degenerative arthritis. In the presence of degenerative arthritic changes there is a persistent crepitation, pain, joint range-of-motion limitation, and concurrent spasm of the muscles of mastication.

In systemic inflammatory arthritis (rheumatoid, psoriatic, anklyosing, gouty, etc.), the TMJ frequently becomes involved. In these pathological conditions there is painful crepitation, limited opening, protrusion, and lateral and rotatory jaw movement, and concurrent masticatory muscle spasm with muscle pain and tenderness.

LABORATORY DIAGNOSIS

Diagnosis of temporomandibular structural disease and impairment to substantiate what appears evident on history and clinical evaluation is enhanced by current diagnostic procedures. Originally routine x-rays were diagnostic only when pathology was advanced. Currently MRI studies have evolved and revealed soft-tissue pathology.[22] Tomograms,[23] CT scanning, contrast studies (arthrographic),[24] and arthroscopic examinations are also available and well-documented. The techniques and diagnostic indication for the choice and interpretation of these diagnostic studies is beyond the scope of this text and will be in the domain of the consultant oral dental specialist.

The temporomandibular joint space (condyle-glenoid) measurement elicited by transcranial images has proven inaccurate.[25] Tomograms are more accurate but require time for evaluation and greater radiation exposure to the patient with no clarity of the soft-tissue component. They are thus not advised for screening. Their accuracy as compared to arthrographic diagnosis has been confirmed.[26] The value of tomography is essentially limited to a determination of the status of the bony condyle vis-à-vis fracture and advanced arthritic changes.

Arthrography has become a well-documented diagnostic procedure in recent decades. This procedure can now be performed with very little discomfort to the patient.[27] Not only can the articular contents be examined, but the dynamics of the joint can be documented.[28] If you are doing a tomogram at the same sitting of arthrography, it is possible to ascertain the bony features of the condyle and the site of the disc. However, these procedures are invasive, with possible allergic reaction to the dye and exposure to radiation. They are also time-consuming and do not give accurate soft-tissue imaging.

CT scanning has emerged as a precise revelation of the site, status, and relationship of the disc as well as the status of the bony structures of the

TMJ articulation.[29] CT scanners are now available in many medical facilities and radiation exposure is not a factor.

Magnetic resonance imaging (MRI) gives greater definition of the soft-tissue structures within the joint, delineating more precisely the position of the disc, early degenerative changes of the disc, and minor tears in the articular cartilage. In recent years there has been voluminous literature regarding MRI studies of the TMJ.[30] The availability of MRI equipment no longer presents a contraindication. MRI is excellent for diagnosis as to indications for surgery, determining the reason for failure of conservative treatment, and possible failure of success after surgery.

Arthroscopy is limited to the upper joint compartment. It confirms disc displacement, articular or disc degeneration, fibrosis or adhesions, pannus formation, glenoid cartilage degeneration, and synovitis. It also allows biopsy of suspect tissue. It is of no value to evaluate the inferior space between the disc and condyle and is an invasive procedure, with all those complications. However, therapeutic procedures are possible in addition to visual diagnosis, and arthroscopy is helpful in treating a locked joint or a recalcitrant unreduced dislocated joint.

Indications for diagnostic procedures are to decide the condition of the disc, whether dislocated, locked, torn, or degenerated, and to determine the condition of the cartilage and ligaments. Treatment obviously demands accurate, precise diagnosis, and often clinical impressions demand confirmation. These tests provide this information.

TREATMENT

When the symptomatic condition is determined to be degenerative arthritis, in essence treatment consists of oral anti-inflammatory medications (NSAID) with all their precautions and contraindications taken into consideration. Local modalities include ice packs to the involved area followed by the local application of heat. Temporary rest of the joint followed by gradual active range-of-motion exercises diminishes the inflammation, decreases the pain, and permits early restoration of pain-free joint motion. Dental assistance for faulty occlusion may be needed as well as a proper orthosis used nocturnally or even daily.

In inflammatory disease that affects the temporomandibular joint, treatment is as indicated for the systemic disease. Rheumatoid arthritis rarely affects the temporomandibular joint, but joint arthralgia in the presence of systemic disease raises that possibility and all local measures to the TMJ are indicated in addition to systemic treatment.

Any occlusion abnormality must be corrected and monitored. Inflammation, weakness, atrophy, and contracture of the masticatory muscles must be addressed. The articular and periarticular tissues must be addressed to ensure adequate opening and physiological motions as well as strength and endurance.

Surgical intervention must be considered when there is persistent, progressive, or even nonresponsive recovery of pain-free function in spite of what is considered appropriate conservative treatment.

TREATMENT OF DISC DERANGEMENT

In the presence of disc derangement with or without locking the vast majority respond to conservative nonsurgical management. In the presence or at least the suspicion of a disc derangement, diagnostic studies (CT scan, MRI, arthroscopy, etc.) may determine the recommended procedure.

In the presence of a click, indicating the possibility of a disc impingement syndrome, there are factors that influence the prognosis and even the preferred treatment. Pain or no pain with the click is a prognostic factor with the presence of pain being more ominous.

The briefer the duration of this clicking history, the more favorable is the response to conservative treatment. The earlier in the opening phase of the jaw motion that the click occurs, the more favorable is the expected response to treatment. If click is reduced by bringing the mandible forward (with orthosis), this is considered a favorable sign especially when there is little distance of jaw position and movement required. If more than 3 to 5 mm of anterior repositioning of the mandible is needed to eliminate the click, the expected response to treatment is less favorable. The earlier the placement of the orthosis from which the patient receives relief, the better is the long-range prognosis.

If the clicking is not painful, treatment is deferred unless the clicking is considered unnacceptable to the patient. The implication is that clicking, per se, is usually reasonably innocuous.[31] However, there is a prevalent opinion that clicking forebodes ultimate degeneration of the disc and/or the cartilage of the joint.[32]

Persistent clicking with pain resulting from mandibular malposition from occlusive disease may favorably respond to repositioning by splint therapy. The benefit from orthosis is noted by the diminution or cessation of the clicking and elimination of the pain. Locking that occurs along with clicking and pain increases the severity of the condition and reduces the favorable response to conservative therapy.

The purpose of occlusal orthosis is essentially to increase the distance between the disc and the condyle, to prevent entrapment of the disc with subsequent damage, and to prevent condylar and genoid articular degeneration. The occlusive device widens the jaw opening and positions the mandible anteriorly or posteriorly, depending on the desired position. The splint needed to open the bite is a flat-plane splint which precedes any

Figure 10–12. Orthosis to open, maintain opening, or reposition the mandible.

In the upper drawing the orthosis (*splint*) is flat-planed to evenly open the bite, realign the teeth, and open the temporomandibular joint (TMJ). This may be therapeutic to open the jaw against the muscular force of the masseter and temporalis muscles.

In the lower drawing the orthosis is angled to reposition the mandible by causing it to move forward and change the bite and the opening of the TMJ. This orthosis may be used to correct. Then there is return to the flat-plane orthosis to maintain the gained TMJ opening.

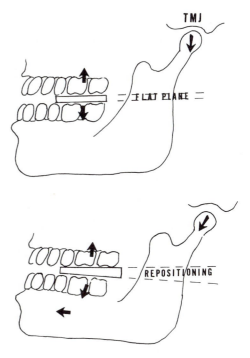

repositioning of the mandible. The amount of opening desired is based on tomography and the elimination of clicking. Both are significantly arbitrary and not precise.

Repositioning of the mandible usually follows the modification of the closed position. Admittedly, some dental therapists reposition the mandible immediately and in conjunction with the opening procedure, but usually repositioning is attempted after several weeks of flat-plane correction. The flat-plane correction also allows time for rehabilitation therapy to the involved masticatory musculature.

From the flat-plane position the orthosis is modified to gradually move the mandible into a protruded position until the clicking is eliminated. (Fig. 10–12). Reposition aims to reduce the space between the condyle in its relationship to the disc. The patient is instructed on gradually moving (anteriorly positioning) the splint in graded degrees, wearing the splint around the clock, and moving the direction of the splint every 2 to 3 weeks.

The angle of repositioning is gradually decreased until the orthosis is again in the flat plane, at which time it is gradually discontinued. The rapidity of each segment of treatment depends upon the experience and judgment of the oral surgeon.

Repositioning the mandible by occlusal appliances is considered reversible in that the original mandibular position recurs after removal of the orthosis. Some structural correction remains, however, so clinicians must keep this factor in mind and not attempt to overcorrect. Correction (rehabilitation) of the masticatory muscles must also be accomplished, as failing to do so may permit deforming forces to remain and affect the occlusion in spite of orthotic correction. It must be remembered that the oral pathology, including the malocclusion, was originally a neuromuscular deficiency and abnormality which, if allowed to persist or recur, will prevent correction and allow recurrence of pain and cause further structural deformity.

The basics of ancillary treatment of TMJ disorder to supplement the orthotic and surgical procedures can be listed as follows:

1. Education of the patient as to the rationale and explanation of purpose
2. Modality implementation for

   • Pain relief
   • Elimination of trigger zones and nodules
   • Increased range of motion
   • Rebalance of agonist and antagonist muscles
   • Increased strength
   • Improved posture

3. Modification of the environment through

   • Education
   • Diminution of stress by means of biofeedback, counseling, and changes in life-style
   • Exercise and diet programs

Masticatory musculature rehabilitation is similar to the basic treatment of fibromyalgia. Decrease of pain is the initial approach with alternating heat and ice applications, gentle massage of the muscles, and gentle passive and active stretching (preceded with vasocoolant spray or ice). Biofeedback may be needed if the patient remains unable to relax the musculature or apprehension cannot be overcome (Fig. 10–13).

The ligaments and muscles that have become restricted in elongation may respond to gradual stretching preceded by local icing and followed by heat (Fig. 10–14). Exercises should be initiated early in the program. Exercise is used to increase passive and active range of motion, strength, endurance, and proprioceptive appreciation. The jaw must be actively and passively opened, protruded, and laterally mobilized. All these motions must gradually be done with assistance then resistance. The tongue must be brought under attention and be "retrained" to avoid the excessive protrusion, which is so prevalent in tense anxious patients.

The palpable trigger points may be eliminated by deep massage, ice, or vasocoolant spray, then stretched. Electrogalvanic stimulation of the trig-

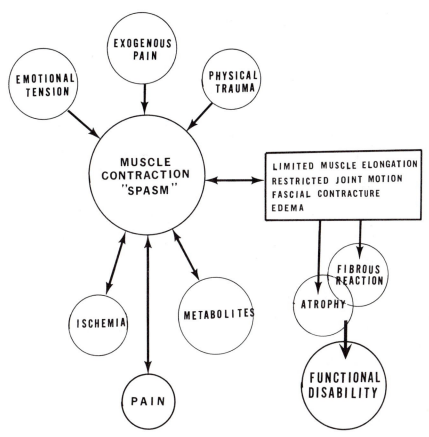

Figure 10–13. Sequence of changes from sustained muscle contraction "spasm."

Sustained muscle contraction described as "spasm" or "tension" is caused by emotional tension, pain stimuli, and trauma. The immediate result is ischemia from compression of the internal blood vessels with accumulation of metabolites and resultant pain which causes further contraction.

The long range sequelae are joint limitation, muscular atrophy, and contracture. Functional disability ultimately results.

ger points has been advocated. If needed, dry needling or injection of the trigger points with saline, an anesthetic agent, and possibly steroids is warranted and often beneficial.

Manipulation of a locked jaw is not the prerogative or expertise of the physical therapist, but when done by a physician, oral surgeon, or orthodontist, it can be preceded and followed by the above physical therapy protocol. The physical therapist, however, can mobilize the mandible (a modification of manipulation), but only if prescribed by the orthodontist or oral surgeon.

It has been estimated that as many as 70 percent of patients with mal-

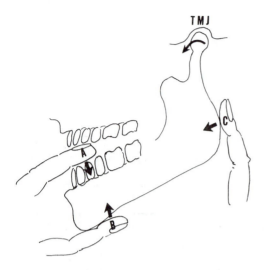

TMJ

Figure 10–14. Passive-active mobilization of the mandible.

(A) Indicates finger inserted into mouth to open the jaw. This stretches the masseter and temporal muscles and their fascia and moves the TMJ anteriorly. (B) The point of resistance to strengthen the muscles that open the jaw. (C) Denotes anterior shear force to protrude the mandible and also anteriorly displace the TMJ.

occlusion have a forward head posture (Fig. 10–15) with an overbite malocclusion (Fig. 10–16).[33] This has been associated with TMJ arthralgia and gradual degeneration as well as degeneration of the cervical vertebral discs. The head, by being forward of the center of gravity weighs relatively more than if the cervical lordosis is minimal and the head is over the center of gravity (Fig. 10–17). In the process facial pain with fatigue and even spasm of the masticatory muscles results. The relationship of posture to malocclusion remains conjectural and is based on the need of parallelism of four planes: the vertical plane, bipupillary plane, plane of the vestibular, and the occlusal (dental) plane (Fig. 10–18). Violation of this parallelism allegedly causes malocclusion.[33] Assuming that there is a postural component to malocclusion, there is definitely a postural component to fibromyalgia and posture must be addressed in treating TMJ disease.

Treating posture remains a difficult problem as there are numerous neurological pathways involved in posture (Fig. 10–19). The basic postural central components reside in the midbrain, pons, and medulla. This center receives input from the periphery (skin, muscles, joints, and ligaments) as well as the labyrinth and neck muscles. Ultimately the innervation of the peripheral muscle affecting the posture occurs through the extrafusal muscle fibers of the total body (Fig. 10–20). Exercises to improve posture (Fig. 10–21) and exercises to decrease the forward head posture (Fig. 10–22) must be supplemented by involving proper posture in every activity of daily living, such as sitting (Fig. 10–23), standing (Fig. 10–24), etc. A weighed object upon the head implements proprioceptive training in erect posture (Figs. 10–25 and 10–26).

The flexibility of the neck soft tissues (muscles ligaments, capsule) must be regained by active and passive exercises done by a therapist, then by the

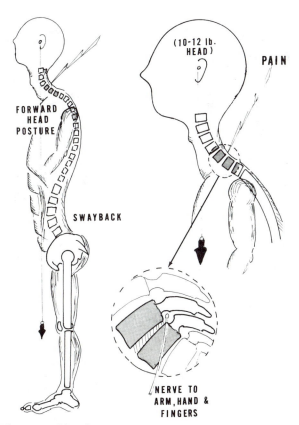

Figure 10–15. Forward head posture.

The head normally should be in direct position over the center of gravity (*plumb line*). If the head is anterior to this line it is called a forward head posture. The head weighing 10–12 pounds places stress upon the neck that has assumed a greater lordosis. The intervertebral foramena are narrowed putting pressure upon the cervical nerve roots. The shoulders (not shown) are in a forward-downward rotation causing strain upon the scapular musculature.

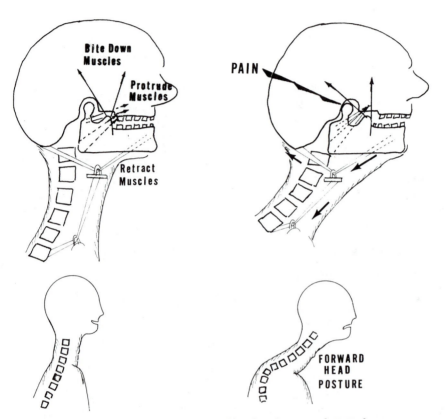

Figure 10–16. Influence of posture upon dental occlusion and TMJ alignment.
The left figure depicts normal posture and its effect upon the bite and TMJ alignment. In the forward head posture (right illustration) the jaw is retracted causing malalignment of the teeth and of the TMJ causing disc deformation, pain, and gradual degenerative changes of the teeth and TMJ. (From Cailliet, R and Gross: The Rejuvenation Strategy. Doubleday, New York, 1987, with permission.)

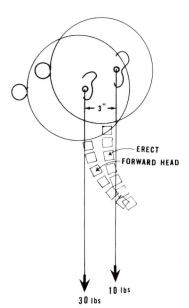

Figure 10–17. Relative weight of the head in the forward head posture.

In the erect posture above the center of gravity the head weighs about 10 pounds. With the head 3 inches ahead of the center of gravity it weighs approximately 30 pounds.

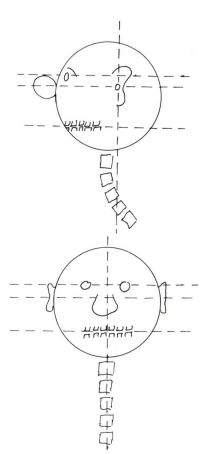

Figure 10–18. Parallel occular, vestibular, and dental alignment related to posture.

To relate posture to dental (and TMJ) alignment a line drawn through the eyes, through the ears (vestibular), and one through the bite should be parallel and perpendicular to the verticle line of the center of gravity.

In a forward head posture these lines (the dental line especially) lose their parallel relationship.

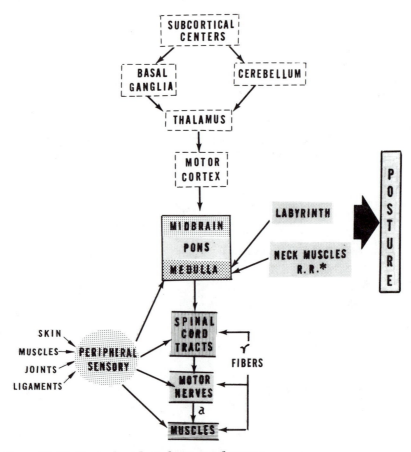

Figure 10–19. Neurophysiological aspects of posture.

Posture is maintained (*controlled*) essentially via pathways of the midbrain which respond to input from the periphery (*sensory*) such as the skin, muscles, joints, and ligaments. The labyrinth and neck muscle righting reflexes (R.R.) also have an input upon the midbrain, medulla, and pons.

The descending pathways through the cord and ultimately the skeletal muscles affect the antigravity components of posture.

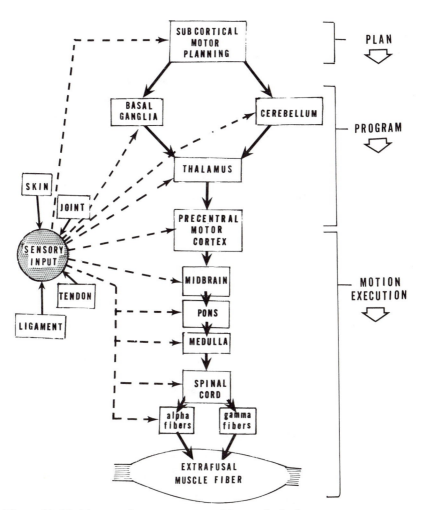

Figure 10–20. Motor pathways to static and kinetic body function.

Upon a chosen motion being decided (plan) and even with static (postural) activities, the action occurs neurophysiologically as indicated until final pathways to the extrafusal muscles are affected. There is a sensory input that coordinates all actions. At the cord level, the degree, rapidity, and duration of the action is monitored via the spindle (intrafusal) alpha and gamma fibers.

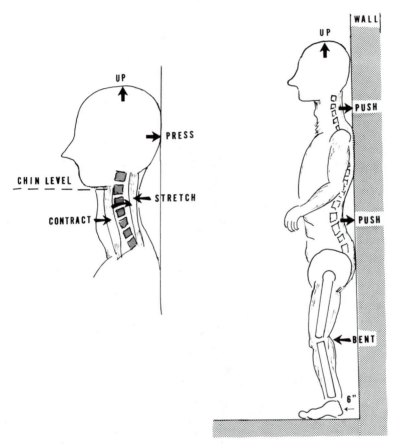

Figure 10–21. Posture exercises and (concept) training.

To maintain an erect posture with proper alignment relative to the center of gravity, the person stands with feet several inches from a wall (6 in). The low back (lumbosacral spine) and the neck (cervical spine) are "pushed" against the wall. This decreases the cervical and lumbar lordosis.

The concept of standing taller *(up)* is initiated. In the left figure the chin is held level, and the neck flexor muscles are contracted which simultaneously stretches the neck extensors.

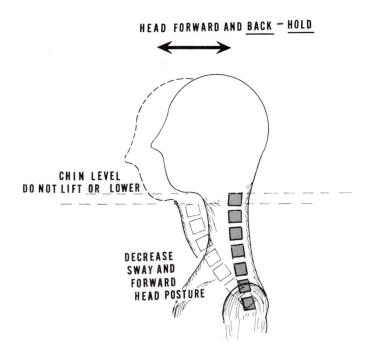

Figure 10–22. Exercise to decrease forward head posture.

Keeping the chin along a level horizontal line the head is pulled back and up, then held and released. This strengthens the neck flexors and stretches the extensors. This exercise which takes but a few minutes can be done frequently during the day and actually be a "break" away from the sustained postures of many daily activities. (From Cailliet, R and Gross: The Rejuvenation Strategy. Doubleday, New York, 1987, with permission.)

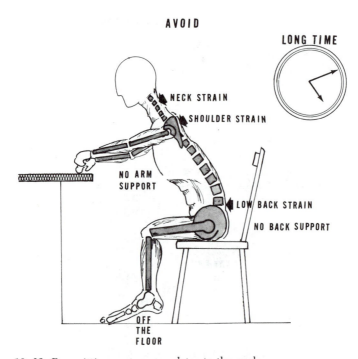

Figure 10–23. Poor sitting posture as relates to the neck.

The sitting posture depicted should be avoided, especially if maintained for long periods of time. In the depicted posture, the head is held in a forward posture causing muscular strain.

Proper sitting posture eliminates all the "No's" listed and encourages frequent "breaks" from the forward head position. (From Cailliet, R and Gross: The Rejuvenation Strategy. Doubleday, New York, 1987, with permission.)

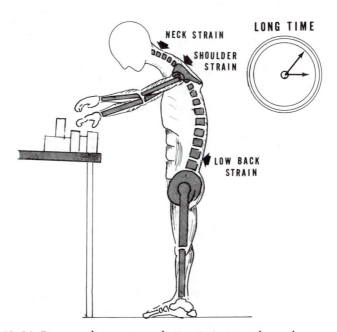

Figure 10–24. Poor standing posture placing strain upon the neck.

The standing posture depicted should be avoided as it places muscular, ligamentous, and disc strain upon the neck and low back as well as the shoulders. Duration of this position should also be moderated. (From Cailliet, R and Gross: The Rejuvenation Strategy. Doubleday, New York, 1987, with permission.)

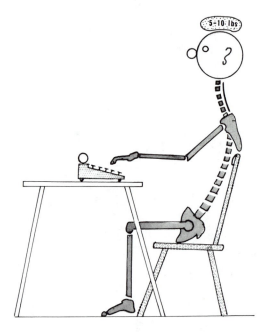

Figure 10–25. Proprioceptive training of erect sitting posture.

With a weight upon the head there is proprioceptive stimulation to keeping the head at the center of gravity. As the head moves forward the weight becomes "heavier" and the muscle reponse (via the mechanoreceptors) is to return to the center of gravity.

patient on a home program (Fig. 10–27). Strength and endurance of the neck muscles must also be regained (Figs. 10–28 and 10–29).

Cervical traction, used frequently as a physical therapy modality to decrease lordosis and elongate the cervical soft tissues, must be used with caution as the traction apparatus can cause pressure upon the TMJ (Fig. 10–30). If traction is used, it should be administered at 20° of flexion in the sitting position (Fig. 10–31) and at the same degree in the reclining position (Fig. 10–32). A collar (Fig. 10–33) may be applied to maintain proper lordosis of the neck, again guarding against excessive mandibular pressure invoked against the TMJ. A night pillow (Fig. 10–34) also assists in controlling the degree of cervical lordosis.

Anti-inflammatory medication is of value, as is the use of antidepressants to increase the endorphin production. Antidepressant medicine for chronic pain is undergoing evaluation. The efficacy of tricyclic medications versus placebo has been established.[34] The antidepressant action of drugs does not correlate with their nociceptive effect. Chlorimipramine, 25 mg, is more effective in serotonin type of pain, whereas nortriptyline, 25 mg, is more active through the noradrenaline system.

The use of transcutaneous nerve stimulation (TENS) is of value for chronic pain. Electrical stimulation of the musculature has been advocated, but the exact neuromuscular physiological effect remains unclear.

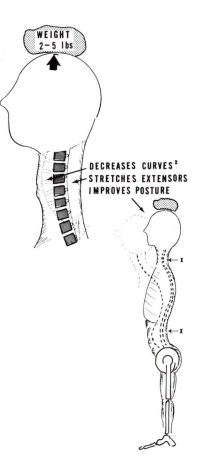

LIFTING

Figure 10–26. Proprioceptive training of erect standing posture.

With a weight upon the head there is proprioceptive stimulation to keep the head at the center of gravity. As the head moves forward, the weight becomes "heavier" and the muscle reponse (via the mechanoreceptors) is to return to the center of gravity.

As in the sitting posture (see Fig. 10–25), this principle can be applied in the standing posture. (From Cailliet, R and Gross: The Rejuvenation Strategy. Doubleday, New York, 1987, with permission.)

NECK STRETCH

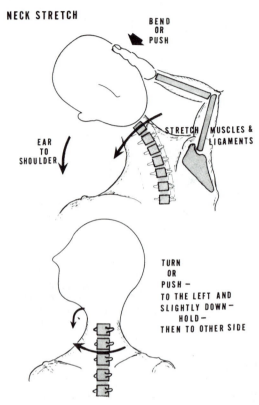

BEND
OR
PUSH

STRETCH MUSCLES &
LIGAMENTS

EAR
TO
SHOULDER

TURN
OR
PUSH −
TO THE LEFT AND
SLIGHTLY DOWN −
HOLD −
THEN TO OTHER SIDE

Figure 10–27. Neck exercises to increase range of motion.

Lateral and rotational range of motion can be attained by manually (self and assisted) stretching. This exercise elongates the muscles, fascia, ligaments and the joint capsules. It can be done frequently taking merely minutes and can be preceded with heat and followed by ice (or vice versa) whichever is the most comfortable. (From Cailliet, R and Gross: The Rejuvenation Strategy. Doubleday, New York, 1987, with permission.)

NECK STRENGTHENING 1

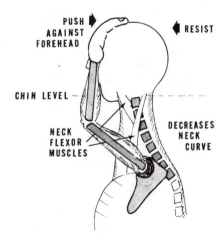

PUSH
AGAINST
FOREHEAD

RESIST

CHIN LEVEL

NECK
FLEXOR
MUSCLES

DECREASES
NECK
CURVE

Figure 10–28. Exercises to strengthen neck muscles 1.

Keeping the chin horizontal (*level*) and applying manual pressure of gradually increasing force strengthens the neck flexors and stretches the neck extensors. (From Cailliet, R and Gross: The Rejuvenation Strategy. Doubleday, New York, 1987, with permission.)

NECK STRENGTHENING 2

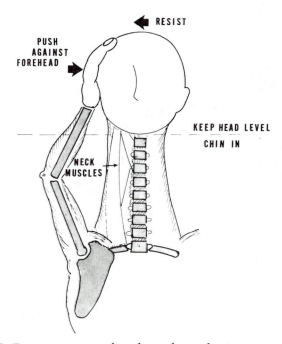

Figure 10–29. Exercises to strengthen the neck muscles 2.

Keeping the chin horizontal (*level*) and applying manual pressure of gradually increasing force strengthens the neck lateral flexors and stretches the opposing lateral neck flexors. (From Cailliet, R and Gross: The Rejuvenation Strategy. Doubleday, New York, 1987, with permission.)

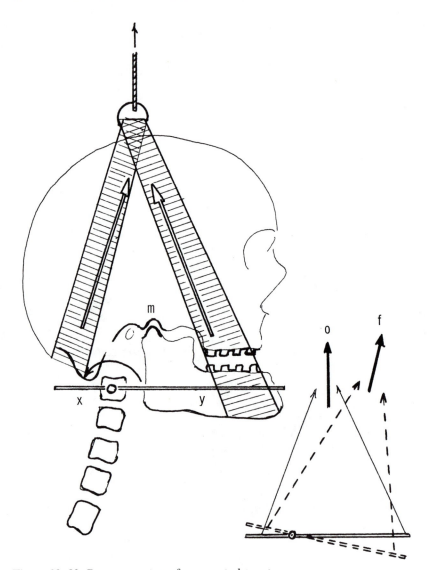

Figure 10–30. Pressure variants from cervical traction.

The halter for applying cervical traction attaches to the occiput (*x*) and under the mandible (*y*). (*m*) indicates the TMJ. If the force is applied in a posterior direction (*o*) there is excessive pressure upon the mandible, whereas if properly applied (20° of flexion) the pressure (*f*) is upon the occiput and the mandible is minimally involved. (From Cailliet, R: Neck and Arm Pain, ed 3. FA Davis, Philadelphia, 1991, p 148, with permission.)

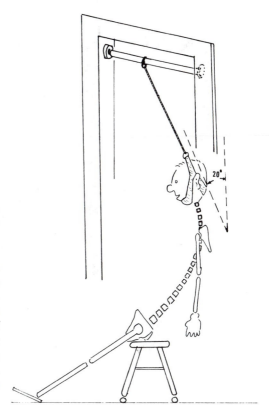

Figure 10–31. Overhead cervical home traction with proper angulation.

At an angle of 20° flexion, there is minimal pressure upon the mandible and most of the force is exerted upon the occiput. The force of traction is determined by the amount of "leaning back" the patient assumes. (From Cailliet, R: Neck and Arm Pain, ed 3. FA Davis, Philadelphia, 1991, p 152, with permission.)

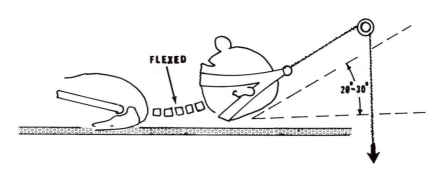

Figure 10–32. Optimal degree of neck flexion in supine cervical traction.

With home supine cervical traction a 20° to 30° flexion must be assured in the daily application of traction. The amount (*force*) of traction is that tolerated by the patient and usually exceeds 10 to 15 pounds. (From Cailliet, R: Neck and Arm Pain, ed 3. FA Davis, Philadelphia, 1991, p 147, with permission.)

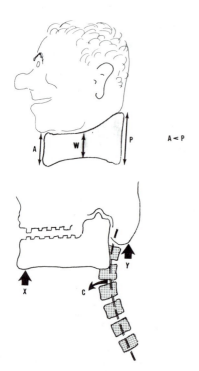

A < P

Figure 10–33. Soft felt cervical collar.

A custom-made (to the precise measurements of the patient) collar must have the anterior width (A) to support the chin and the posterior width (P) to elevate the occiput. The lateral width (W) fits under the angle of the mandible.

A felt cervical collar does not distract the head and neck; it essentially maintains and supports the head in a horizontal position and thus decreases the cervical lordosis. (From Cailliet, R: Neck and Arm Pain. FA Davis, Philadelphia, 1991, p 93, with permission.)

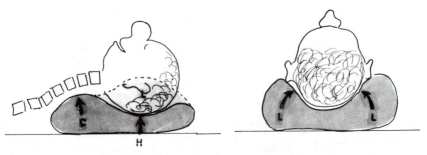

Figure 10–34. Sleeping pillow to maintain physiological lordosis.

There are numerous types of pillows that support the head and neck in a comfortable physiological lordosis. The portion behind the head (H) is for comfort and the width of the pillow behind the neck (C) assures the degree of lordosis. There are lateral elevations (L) that maintain the position of the head and prevent nocturnal rotation. (From Cailliet, R: Neck and Arm Pain, ed 3. FA Davis, Philadelphia, 1991, p 153, with permission.)

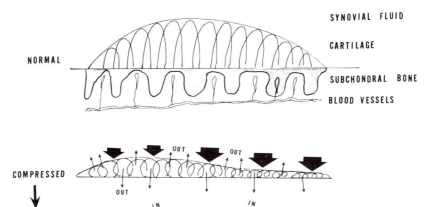

Figure 10–35. Normal cartilage nutrition and lubrication.

The upper illustration depicts the cartilage with its coiled collagen fibers, the synovial fluid, the subchondral bone, and end blood vessels.

When mechanically compressed (*large arrows*) fluid is compressed out into the joint space which contains lubricating substances. There is also fluid exchange with the capillaries of the subchondral bone (*small arrows*).

When pressure is released the matrix of the cartilage 'imbibes' the synovial fluid. The imbibition acts to nutritionally supply the matrix. The compression lubricates the joint. (From Cailliet, R: Knee Pain and Disability, ed 2. FA Davis, Philadelphia, 1983, p 91, with permission.)

DEGENERATIVE ARTHRITIC CHANGES OF THE TMJ

A major purpose of correct occlusion is to maintain the integrity of the temporomandibular joint as well as preserving the integrity of the teeth. The latter is to prevent dental problems, a topic that is beyond the scope of this dissertation, although face and head pain are elicited by dental problems. The preservation of TMJ integrity is to avoid the ultimate degenerative articular changes of the glenoid fossa and the condyle. Both are covered with cartilage, which is an avascular tissue that receives its nutrition from the capsular blood vessels and diffusion from the bone end vessels.

So long as the collagen coils within the cartilage matrix remain intact the inhibitory aspects of the cartilage maintain normal nutrition and therefore normal function—compression (shock absorption) and lubrication of the joint (Fig. 10–35).

The joint space may be too narrow because of a gradual loss of the

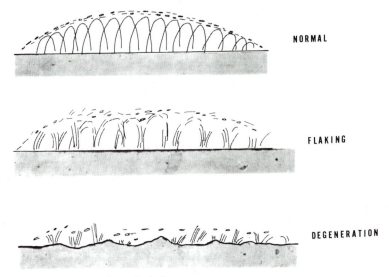

Figure 10–36. Stages of cartilage degeneration.

Normal cartilage exposed to excessive compression and shear forces initially undergoes "flaking" in which the coiled ends of the collagen fibers are damaged and can no longer mechanically act to oppose compression and to recoil for imbibition. The matrix expels fragments of the damaged cartilage into the joint.

With further degeneration the coiled collagen fibers are further damaged, as is the matrix, and there are areas of denuded subchondral bone. (From Cailliet, R: Knee Pain and Disability, ed 2. FA Davis, Philadelphia, 1983, p 91, with permission.)

intervening meniscus. In this case, there may be excessive shear on the cartilage, causing the outer surface of the cartilage to flake (Fig. 10–36). The disrupted collagen coils no longer permit compression and expansion of the cartilage; this leads to gradual degeneration and ultimate denuding of the underlying bone. The degenerated cartilage exposes the underlying bone, resulting in pain and further diminution of motion. Limited motion results in diminished cartilage nutrition. A vicious cycle of progressive degenerative arthritis is thus evoked and becomes irreversible.

MANIPULATION OF A LOCKED JAW

Manual manipulation of a locked jaw, if acute, may be an office procedure depending on the experience and facilities of the practitioner. The patient needs to be premedicated with a muscle relaxant, sedative, or nerve block. Intra-articular injection of an anesthetic may be utilized. If the jaw is chronically blocked, the procedure should be performed by an oral surgeon in a surgical facility to ensure the maintenance of an adequate airway and to avoid respiratory cardiovascular complications. After manipulation an orthosis may be required to maintain the opened temporomandibular joint. The patient must be followed by daily physical therapy to maintain or regain the acquired range of motion and to decrease the inflammation and muscular spasm that preceded manipulation and has been aggravated by the manipulation.

SURGICAL INTERVENTION

In an uncorrectable meniscus displacement, significant tear of the meniscus. Arthroscopic intervention for diagnostic purposes is available, and while the arthroscope is in the joint space the disc can be mobilized, resected, or restored. The extent of surgical intervention will depend upon the significance of the damage found and the expertise and experience of the surgeon[35] in correcting or modifying the pathology.

Open joint surgery has been advocated and utilized permitting a longer period and greater exposure of the joint than does arthroscopic intervention. With this exposure repositioning of the meniscus (meniscorrhaphy) and plication correction is facilitated. Total or partial meniscectomy is advocated by some, with definitive indications based on the experience of the surgeon.[36] Attempts have been made to replace a disc with an implant, but experience with this procedure is limited and the results have been variable. In the presence of a normal intact joint cartilage of the glenoid and the fossa, a partial or total meniscectomy, followed by comprehensive rehabilitation, is advised.

REFERENCES

1. Headache Classification Committee of the Internal Headache Society. Classification and diagnostic criteria for headache disorders, cranial neuralgias, and facial pain. Cephalalgia (Suppl)8:1–96, 1988.
2. MacConnail, MA: Studies in the mechanics of synovial joints. Ir J Med Sci 21:223, 1946.
3. Cailliet, R: Mechanics of joints. In Licht, E (ed): Arthritis and Physical Medicine. Elizabeth Licht, New Haven, 1969.
4. Cailliet, R: Mechanics of joints. In Cailliet, R.: Shoulder Pain. ed 3. FA Davis, Philadelphia, 1991, pp 4–9.
5. McNeill, C (ed): Craniomandibular Disorders: Guidelines for Evaluation, Diagnosis and Management. Quintessence, Chicago, 1990.
6. Harness, DM, Donion, WC, and Eversole, LR: Myogenic, TMJ, internal derangement and atypical facial pain patients. Am Assoc Dent Res 1078:316, 1989.
7. Plunket, GAJ and West, VC: J Craniomand Pract 6:320–326, 1988.
8. Katzberg, RW, et al: J Prosthet Dent 49:250–254, 1983.
9. Rugh, JD and Harlan, J: Adv Neurol 49:329–341, 1988.
10. Sheikoleslam, A, Holmgren, K, and Riise, C: J Oral Rehabil 13:137–145, 1986.
11. Catesby, WJ and Rugh, JD: Sleep 11:172–181, 1988.

12. Clark, GT and Adler, RC: JADA 110:743–750, 1985.
13. Pierce, CJ and Gale, EN: J Dent Res 11:172–181, 1988.
14. Graff-Radford, SB: Oromandibular disorders and headache. A critical appraisal. In Mathew, N (ed): Neurological Clinics. WB Saunders, Philadelphia, 1991.
15. Costen, JB: A syndrome of ear and sinus problems dependent on disturbed function of the temporomandibular joint. Ann Otol Rhinol Laryngol 43:1–15, 1934.
16. Carette, S, McCain, GA, Bell, DA, and Fam, AG: A double blind study of amitriptyline versus placebo in patients with primary fibrositis. Arthr Rheum 29:655–659, 1986.
17. Hagberg, C: Electromyography and bite force studies of muscular function and dysfunction in masticatory muscles. Swedish Dental J, Umea (Suppl)37:1–64, 1986
18. Eversole, LR and Machado, L: JADA 110:69–79, 1985.
19. Scott, DS: Myofascial pain-dysfunction syndrome: A psychobiological perspective. J Behav Med 4:451–463, 1981.
20. Salter, MW, Brooke, R, Mersky, H, Fichter, GF, and Kapusionyk, DH: Is the temporomandibular pain and dysfunction syndrome a disorder of the mind? Pain 17:151–166, 1987.
21. Salter, MW, Brooke, RI, and Mersky, H: Temporomandibular pain and dysfunction syndrome: The relationship of clinical and psychological data to outcome. J Behav Med 9:97–109, 1986.
22. Helms, CA, et al: J Craniomand Pract 2:220–224, 1984.
23. Petrilli, A and Gurley, JE: JADA 20:218–224, 1939.
24. Katzberg, RW, et al: AJR 132:949–955, 1980.
25. Liedberg, J, Robin, M, and Westesson, PI: Acta Odontol Scand 43:53–58, 1985.
26. Ronquillo, HI, et al: J Craniomand Dis 2(55):1–24, 1988.
27. Donlon, WC, Truta, MP, and Eversole, LR: J Oral Maxillofac Surg 42:544–545, 1984.
28. Farrar, WB and McCarty, WI: J Prosthet Dent 41:548–555, 1979.
29. Helms, CA, et al: Radiology 145:719–723, 1982.
30. Kaplan, P, et al: Radiology 165:177–178, 1987.
31. Lundh, H, Westesson, PL, and Kopp, S: Oral Surg 3:530–533, 1987
32. Greene, CS and Laskin, DM: JADA 117:461–465, 1988.
33. Rocabado, M, Johnston, BE, and Blakney, MG: Physical therapy and dentistry: An overview. Phys Ther 1(1):47–49, 1983.
34. Panerai, AE, et al: A randomized, within-patient crossover, placebo-controlled trial on the efficacy and tolerability of the tricyclic antidepressants chlorimipramine and nortriptyline in central pain. Acta Neurol Scand 82:34–38, 1990.
35. Sanders, B, Murakami, K-J, and Clark, GT: Diagnostic and surgical arthroscopy of the temporomandibular joint. WB Saunders, Philadelphia, 1989.
36. Kiehn, CH: Meniscectomy for internal derangements of the TMJ. Am J Surg 364, Mar, 1952.

CHAPTER 11

Neurophysiological-Psychological Basis for the Management of Head-Face Pain

Pain is a warning signal that helps to protect the body from tissue damage. The sensation of pain originates from the activation of nociceptive primary afferents by intense thermal, mechanical, or chemical stimuli. These nociceptor sites are small, free nerve endings, and the noniceptive stimuli are numerous.

Two decades ago it was thought that tissue damage and injury produced increased sensitization of the peripheral nociceptors and that this was the basis for hyperalgesia at the site of injury.[1] It was also thought that peripheral injury increased excitability in the spinal dorsal horn.[2] If the excitability of the injured tissues of the periphery was diminished, it seemed apparent that the excitability of the central spinal horn could also be diminished and thus pain could be diminished.[3,4]

Chemical mediators are released or synthesized from the damaged tissue. When these mediators accumulate in sufficient quantity, they activate the receptors. Among these chemical mediators are phospholipids, which break down from arachidonic acid to form prostaglandin E (Fig. 11–1). Inflammatory mediators called leukotrines are also liberated from trauma. These leukotrienes do not undergo the same breakdown sequence of arachidonic acid and are not influenced by NSAID medications. Trauma also causes a breakdown of blood platelets. This releases serotonin, which acts

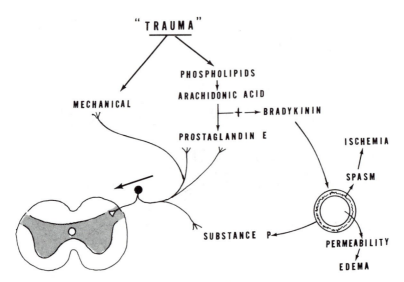

Figure 11–1. Nociceptive substances liberated from trauma.

Regardless of the type of trauma, the traumatized tissue liberates breakdown products from phospholipids into arachidonic acid and ultimately prostaglandins.

The trauma also affects the blood vessels causing spasm, edema, and liberation of platelets that breakdown to free serotonin and substance P. Other kinins and toxic substances are nociceptive products that irritate nerve endings causing ultimate pain.

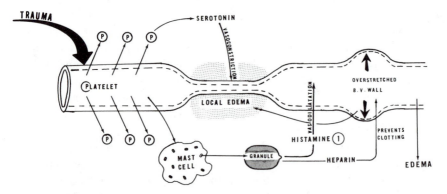

Figure 11–2. Schematic concept of vasochemical sequelae of trauma.

The microhemorrhage or macrohemorrhage releases serotonin which causes vasoconstriction and releases mast cells. The granules of these mast cells release histamine, which causes vasodilation with resultant edema.

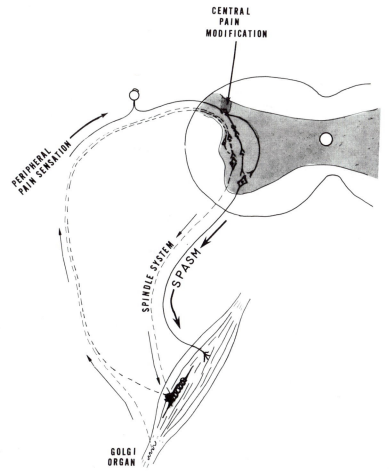

Figure 11–3. Neural pattern for production of spasm resulting from pain (postulated).
The nociceptive impulses ascending to the dorsal horn become modified at the layers of Rexed. A mononeural reflex.

as a vasoconstrictor and causes local edema (Fig. 11–2). The resultant muscle spasm that locally accompanies trauma is possibly mediated through a neural pattern, wherein the nociceptor impulses emanating through the dorsal root ganglia (DRG) send impulses via neuronal connections to the anterior horn cell (AHC), with resultant muscular contraction (Fig. 11–3). The nociceptor stimuli can emanate from the skin, blood vessels, joint capsules, ligaments, and muscles (Fig. 11–4). The muscle thus involved as recipient of the nociceptive reaction becomes an initiator of nociception, setting up a vicious cycle of painful muscle spasm which in turn becomes the nociceptor site of pain.

There are many chemical nociceptive mediators other than histamine,

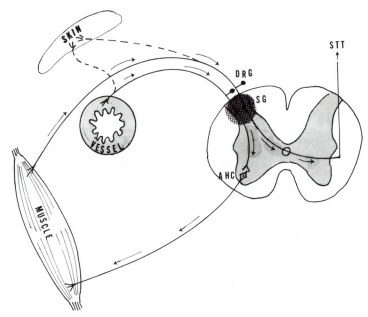

Figure 11–4. Neural patterns emanating from skin, blood vessels, and muscles causing "spasm" (a vicious cycle).

The muscle held in sustained contraction ("spasm") creates nociceptive substances that ascend through the dorsal root ganglia *(DRG)* into the substantia gelatinosum *(SG)* that traverses to the spinothalamic tracts *(STT)* to the thalamus. A branch innervates the anterior horn cell *(AHC)* which causes further extrafusal muscle contraction. Muscle inflammation (ischemia, lactic acid, etc.) becomes the site of sustained nociception.

substance P, and the many leukotrienes that are being reported almost weekly in the research literature.

Fig. 11–5 shows the sensory nociceptive fibers entering the dorsal horn.[5-7] The dorsal horn is divided into five lamina, which were originally combined in Lissauer's tract.[8] Each lamina has a specific task in differentiating the afferent pain inputs. Areas of the dorsal horn of the spinal cord are subserved by both somatic-sensory and visceral-autonomic fibers.

Lamina V responds to both cutaneous and visceral nerve stimulation.[9] These connections between somatic and sympathetic (autonomous) systems are of increasing clinical significance in determining the neurological pathways of pain.

Strong cutaneous stimulation can affect the activity of preganglionic autonomic neurons in the lateral horns of the spinal cord.[10] Two types of nociceptor (fast and slow) have terminals in lamina V, although most terminate in lamina I to IV. Sympathetic discharges, fired over a long period of time, can initiate somatic muscular contraction. The resultant sustained

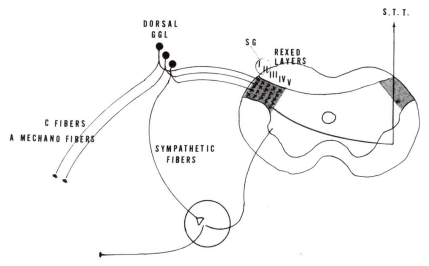

Figure 11–5. Sensory fibers entering the dorsal root.

The sensory C fibers, mechano A fibers, and sympathetic sensory afferent fibers enter the dorsal horn into the cord gray matter. The dorsal horn is divided into numerous (IV or more layers of Rexed) where the main sensory fibers enter layers of Rexed I and II, which constitute the substantia gelatinosum (*S.G.*). Sensory impulses traverse the cord to ascend in the spinothalamic tracts (*S.T.T.*).

One third of unmyelinated C fibers are considered to enter the dorsal column via the motor roots of the anterior horn (not shown in illustration).

muscular tension results in ischemic myalgia, which in turn becomes a site of nociception.

Most (80 percent) of the afferent peripheral nerves which transmit the impulses that will ultimately evoke the sensation of pain are unmyelinated nerves (C fibers). These fibers conduct very slowly and enter the dorsal column and immediately synapse with the neurons crossing through the anterior commissure to ascend to the thalamus via the spinothalamic tracts to the thalamus (Fig. 11–6). All of the remaining sensory nerves that can conduct noxious stimuli are myelinated nerves of small diameter. The larger-diameter myelinated sensory nerves respond to innocuous stimuli such as mechanical, touch, temperature, and proprioceptive stimuli. Recently, anatomists have demonstrated that approximately one third of all afferent small-diameter unmyelinated C fibers enter the cord through the anterior route.[11] These fibers also have their cell bodies in dorsal root ganglia. This fact may well explain the mechanism of muscle pain, wherein ascending motor fibers to the extrafusal fibers also carry ascending sensory fibers.

Pain sensation is also transmitted through neurons of the α-delta neurons that also synapse in the dorsal horn of the cord and proceed superiorly through the lateral spinothalamic tracts to the thalamus. Several sensations

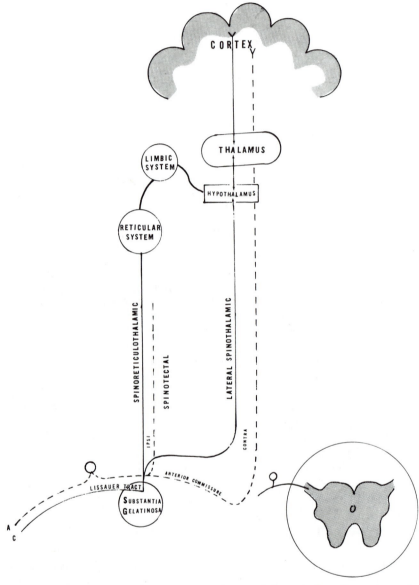

Figure 11–6. Major ascending sensory pathways of the spinal cord carrying pain-mediating fibers.

The two major pathways for pain transmission are the spinothalamocortical system that has spatiotemporal localization and the spinoreticulothalamic system that has no localization but is involved in emotional (limbic) and avoidance reaction.

Both ascend through the substantia gelatinosum of Lissauer's tract (now termed layers of Rexed I and II). The reticular system associates with the hypothalamic-limbic system and relates emotions with the sensation of pain.

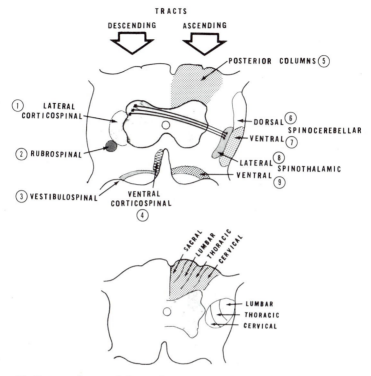

Figure 11–7. Ascending and descending tracts of the spinal cord.

Besides the spinothalamic tracts *(8) (9)* there are numerous tracts that carry motor, sensory, and coordinating functions. All are needed for function but not all transmit sensation nor pain.

are transmitted via the spinothalamic tracts, of which an estimated 54 percent are pain sensations and 46 percent are temperature sensations.

The unmyelinated C fibers are more numerous in the peripheral sensory fibers than are the α-delta fibers and proceed cephalad in a different manner. The α-delta fibers have essentially one neuronal synapse whereas the entering C fibers synapse with numerous short intersegmental neurons that ascend cephalad through multiple ascending system (MAS) synaptic pathways. Some ascending paths are in the dorsal columns as well as in the anterolateral columns (Fig. 11–7).

The speed of impulse determines a selectivity of the type of pain transmitted. The α-delta fibers transmit faster and carry "sharp" pain whereas the C fibers are slower and carry a "dull" longer-lasting pain. As this text considers head and face pain, the trigeminal nerve consists of fibers that carry sharp pain and travels toward the thalamus as part of the lateral lemniscus and trigeminal lemniscus, ending in the ventrobasal nucleus of the thalamus.

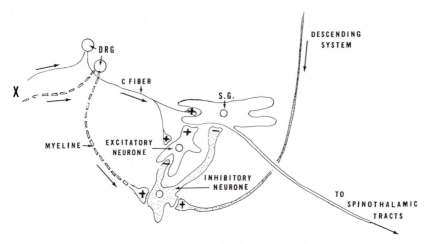

Figure 11–8. Nociceptive transmission to the dorsal horn of the cord.

A schematic version of nociceptive transmission to the dorsal horn is presented. X is the noxious stimulus that is transmitted through afferent C fibers and myelinated large-diameter fibers. In the substantia gelatinosum (S.G.) of the dorsal horn the impulses go to and activate (+) the transmission cell of the S.G. Impulses from the myelinated fibers activate the inhibitory neurones (−) which modulate the projection cell. Ultimately the impulses are transmitted to the lateral spinothalamic tracts where they ascend to the thalamus. The descending tracts also modulate the impulses arriving at the transmission cells.

The ascending fibers of the MAS synapse with neurons of the reticular system in the midbrain (see Fig. 1–16), which processes diffuse fibers from all cranial nerves and upper motor-sensory brain systems including the cortex. The reticular system also relates to the hypothalamus and limbic systems, which again interpose the emotions to the sensory system.

The thalamus divides into two major systems: the MAS and the ventrobasal. The latter consists of the lateral and posterior nuclei, which receive the fast conducting impulses. This system is topographically organized, meaning that the sensations received relate to specific points of the face, head, and body. The neurons of the other system receiving the impulses of the MAS are not specifically organized. These latter fibers radiate to the general cerebral cortex and the limbic system, which is concerned with memory and emotions.

The afferent fibers that enter the dorsal horn relay the information of the nociception (Fig. 11–8). These are termed projection (transmission) fibers. This information is complex and originates from nociception and nonnociception, therefore carrying other innocuous sensations. In the dorsal root, besides unmyelinated sensory fibers carrying nociceptor impulses, there are afferent myelinated fibers, which enter the dorsal horn of the cord carrying inhibitory impulses (Fig. 11–8). The large myelinated fibers that enter the dorsal horn essentially moderate (inhibit) the nociceptive impulses transmitted via the unmyelinated C fibers. This explains the efficacy of TENS, which is carried by the large myelinated fibers.

If the large myelinated fibers are interrupted, the nociceptive fiber impulses are uninhibited, causing the pain to be more severe. This indicates that a peripheral stimulus, both noxious and innocuous, reaches the dorsal horn and undergoes modulation at that site. As a noxious stimulus is transmitted via all the sensory fibers—unmyelinated and myelinated—these sensations must be modulated at the cord level. The concept of pain modulation has been termed the Wall-Melzak gate theory (Fig. 11–9). The modulation occurs at the dorsal horn level but now is also known to occur at the dorsal root level and at more central levels in the midbrain area.

The physiology of afferent nociceptors has been enhanced by the discovery of the chemistry of transmission. These chemical substances released by damaged tissue cells at the site of injury and considered to be the initiators of pain are termed *algogenic*. They have been analyzed as being neuropeptides. As shown in Fig. 11–2, at the site of injury there occurs edema, vasoconstriction, and then vasodilitation with resultant pain. As a result of these local changes at the site of injury (inflammation) polypeptides termed kinins are liberated. Prostaglandins are also involved at this tissue site. Similar algogenic substances are being discovered at each level of nerve and cord transmission.

The chemical modulators of pain have been termed endorphins (enkephalins), which are endogenous opioid substances synthesized by nerve cells. They have their effect at numerous sites along the nerve pathways of the sensory system. These enkephalins have been found in nerve cells at the midbrain, medulla, spinal cord, and dorsal root ganglia. The first neuropeptides discovered were leucine and methionine enkephalin. Many more have been found since.

Finding the chemical basis for pain relief from these kinins has clarified, to a large degree, the fundamental basis for the pain-relieving action of narcotics like morphine sulphate, meperidine hydrochloride, Percodan, etc. These narcotics essentially mimic the action of the intrinsic endorphins at the numerous synapses of the central nervous system.

The chemical mediators of pain in the central nervous system have been studied; currently identified are amino acids (glutaminic acid and aspartic acid), neuropeptides, and monoamines. The amino acids act upon receptor sites at the dorsal horn.[11] The hyperactivity of the central receptors can be initiated by electrical stimulation of C fibers, which apparently occurs via these N-methyl-D-aspartate (NMDA) receptors.[12] The hyperexcitability can be prevented by administration of D-CPP NMDA antagonists.[13] Ketamine, a noncompetitive NMDA antagonist, has been considered effective in reducing postoperative pain.[13] Similar drugs to ketamine are now being sought, and other sites than NMDA are also being researched.

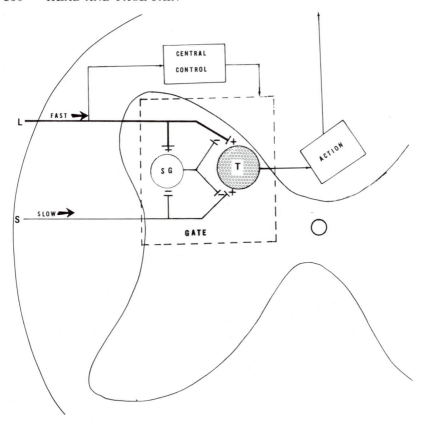

Figure 11–9. "GATE" theory of Wall and Melzak.

The gray area is the dorsal horn region of the cord (The layers of Rexed of which regions I and II are the substantia gelatinosa SG). The sensory fibers carrying noci-ceptor *(C neuron slow pain)* impulses activate (+) the SG, which then proceed to the fibers ascending to the reticular formation via spinoreticulothalamic tracts and the spinothalamic tracts *(STT)* to the thalamus and reticular system. These impulses ultimately are interpreted as "pain."

Neuron fast fibers and mechano A neuron fast fibers enter the dorsal root and stimulate inhibitory (−) fibers *(I)* that modulate the severity of the slower acting C neuron fibers. The gray area is the "gate" area. (From Cailliet, R: Soft Tissue Pain and Disability, ed 2. FA Davis, Philadelphia, 1988, p 25, with permission.)

Other neurochemical mediators from tissue damage have been found to initiate hyperexcitability of the central nervous system, and their antag-onists afford promise in the future of pain management. Among the numerous endorphins can be added norepinephrine and serotonin.

There is now evidence that NMDA plays a major role in several types of seizures developing into epilepsy. The role of NMDA in migraine, migraine variants, and cluster headaches remains unclear. The acute pain experienced by the patient suffering with migraine, migraine variants, cluster headache, trigeminal neuralgia, and other neuralgias have been discussed in Chapters 2, 3, 4, and 5.

Chronic pain in the head and face are the most common sites of chronic pain and form a diverse group of patients. The International Association for the Study of Pain (IASP) has classified this patient category according to five site axes: (1) site of pain, (2) physiological system, (3) temporal pattern and recurrence, (4) intensity and duration, and (5) etiology.[14]

Acute pain relates to recurrent pain and ultimately can become chronic pain. Any pain that lasts longer than 3 months is considered chronic pain, but that arbitrary time distinction is now varied. Some pain states are considered chronic in shorter periods of time and some pains lasting longer are arbitrarily considered but not so labeled.

Before considering how acute or recurrent pain becomes chronic pain, we should review acute and recurrent pain. Acute pain occurs when there has been nociceptive stimulation of the nerve endings of nerves that ascend to the dorsal horn of the cord through the dorsal root ganglion. The concept that pain is a specific sensation and that its intensity is proportional to the degree of tissue (noxious) damage is no longer tenable. Pain is a sensory experience influenced by attention, expectancy, learning, anxiety, fear, and distraction.[15]

The selection and modification of the sensory component of noxious transmission is neurologically accepted (Fig. 11–6), but the receptive system of the dorsal horn and every higher level is directly influenced by expectancy, attention, learning, anxiety, and fear (among others) (Fig. 11–10).

Emotions affect the peripheral ventral mechanism of pain transmission through the limbic system, which then affects the descending tracts to the dorsal horn of the cord and ascending tracts to the thalamus (lateral spinothalamic tracts and spinoreticulothalamic tracts), and finally the cortex (Fig. 11–11). These emotions are basically of three categories: (1) perceptual information locating the site of the noxious insult, (2) motivational tendency indicating the need for reaction by the patient, and (3) cognitive information which is based on previous information.[15] The perceptual information implies the significance of the tissue damaged and its sequelae. The motivational information causes fight or flight, and the cognitive information involves previous experiences and their sequelae. Anxiety, anger, depression, etc., are all involved. Treatment of chronic pain must consider and attack all these sites.

Pain is modulated by chemical substances which are secreted by nerve cells (endorphins) that can be experimentally blocked by naloxone. The release of nociceptive substances that initiate ultimate pain and the resultant relief by endorphins can be blocked by naloxone. This has shed much light on causation of pain by trauma, stress, anxiety, and depression, and clarified the inhibition of pain within the CNS.

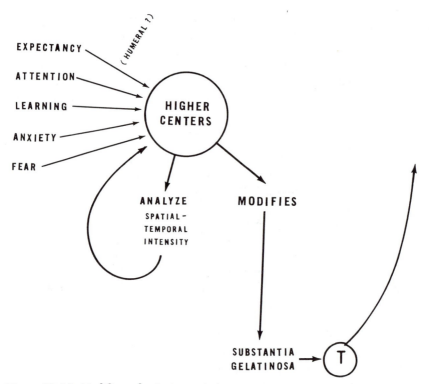

Figure 11–10. Modifiers of pain transmission.

The higher centers which interpret pain as a sensation are modified by humerous factors that involve expectation, attention, learning, anxiety, and fear. These factors modify and analyze sensation at the gray matter level *(SG)* of the cord *(T)* and at the thalamus hypothalamus and the cervical cortex.

Chronic pain has too long been viewed by the medical profession as an organic-psychogenic dichotomy. We must now consider it to be a complex synthesis of biological, psychological, behavioral, and neurohormonal-chemical factors.

The role of the autonomic nervous system in the realm of pain is now also becoming more apparent. The functional anatomy of the autonomic system is well documented (Fig. 11–12). Its clinical significance in the production of pain is being further evaluated, especially in conditions of reflex sympathetic dystrophy (RSD).[16] RSD is not significantly prominent in head and face pain, but certain autonomic aspects of this condition are probably greater than has been perceived.

Neuronal (facial, trigeminal, etc.) function is considered to be axonal transport of protein, which is conveyed along the length of the nerve fiber (Fig. 11–13). This transported protein tissue is highly dependent upon adequate blood supply. Pressure upon the nerve axon with concurrent impaired

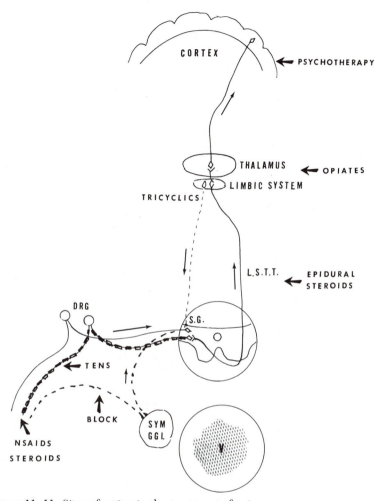

Figure 11–11. Sites of action in the treatment of pain.

The aspirin, steroid, and nonsteroidal site of action is at the peripheral area of noxious tissue injury. The myelinated nerves respond to TENS and the sympathetic nerves transmitting pain respond to sympathetic blocks. The ascending tract: Lateral spinothalamic tracts *(L.S.T.T.)* are the site of epidural steroids and anaesthetic agents and the thalamus, the site of opiates. Psychotherapy influences the interpretation of pain at the cortex level. Tricyclics and other antidepressants effect the descending tracts to the dorsal root: substantia ganglia *(S.G.)*. DRG is the dorsal root ganglion which is effected also by tricyclics.

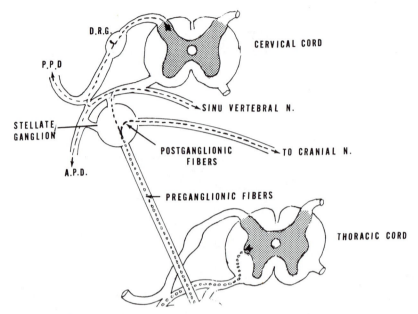

Figure 11–12. Sympathetic nervous system.

The (white) preganglionic fibers originate from the intermediolateral horn cells of the thoracic cord and ascend to the stellate ganglia where they synapse with the postganglionic *(gray)* fibers.

There are sympathetic fibers that accompany the somatic nerves within the anterior primary divisions *(A.P.D.)* and the posterior primary divisions *(P.P.D.)* of nerve roots.

The sensory nerves enter the dorsal column via the dorsal root ganglia *(D.R.G.)*. The sympathetic nerves carry pain *(paresthesia)* sensation and are motor to the blood vessels, sweat glands, and pilatory glands.

blood flow impairs axonal transportation. A nerve so constricted reacts by collateral branching.[17] These branchings become α-adrenogenic receptors,[18] resulting in numerous abnormal ectopic pacemakers that bombard the central nervous system, causing interference with normal processing of sensory information. The central nervous system, already hypersensitive and hyperreactive from previous bombardment from the unmyelinated sensory nerves, overreacts from excessive adrenaline impulses. The excessive peripheral adrenalin production[19] and the excessive central accumulation enhances persistence of pain. This central aberrant sensory processing produces the sensation of pain (paresthesia) (Fig. 11–14).

The psychological aspects of pain are well accepted, but the neural-psychological-humeral aspects remain obscure. Excessive norepinephrine release from anxiety, stress, and fear are considered prominent.

Psychological stress over a long period of time causes stimulation of the

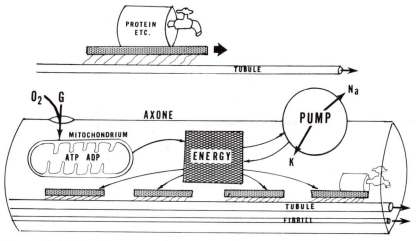

Figure 11–13. Axoplasmic neural transport: a theory.

The *flow* of protein and other derivatives begins with entry of glucose (G) into the fiber. Glycolysis and phosphorylation occur (O_2) in the mitochondria through metabolism of adenosine-triphosphate (ATP), which creates the energy to the sodium pump. This pump regulates balance of sodium (N_a) and potassium (K) and determines nerve activity.

The transport *filaments* (F) move along the axon by occillation and carry the nutritive protein elements along the nerve pathway. (Data from Ochs, S: Axoplasmic transport: A basis for neural pathology.) (From Cailliet, R: Shoulder Pain, ed 3. FA Davis, Philadelphia, 1991, p 229, with permission.)

hypothalamus via the nucleus reticularis paragigantocellularis (RPGC) in the medulla.[20] From the medulla there are many projections to the hypothalamus, especially the paraventricular nuclei (PVN).[21] The PVN contains neurons that release vasopressin and oxytocin, which enter the posterior pituitary gland. There is chemical interplay between the posterior and the anterior pituitary glands with a release of corticotropin hormone and ACTH. This is termed *preponderence of sympathetic release*. The resultant hypothalamic-pituitary-adrenal (HPA) axis is the neurological-hormonal response to stress.[22–24]

In many painful states there is hypersensitivity of the involved tissues, apparently mediated through mechanoreceptors in areas already hypersensitized. This is true of many facial pains, where a mere touch is rejected. A similar aspect of this has emerged in RSD.[25] The theory is that repeated impulses from nociceptor C fibers impinging upon the dorsal horn form a hypersensitivity in the region. The initial trauma causing noxious reaction upon the C-nociceptor fibers proceed through their dorsal root ganglia and impinge upon the dorsal column layer of Rexed I and II (Fig. 11–15). These bombard the adjacent area of the dorsal root. The wide dynamic range (WDR) neurons, having become hypersensitive, accept impulses from mechanoreceptor fibers emanating from myelinated fibers carrying innocuous sensations

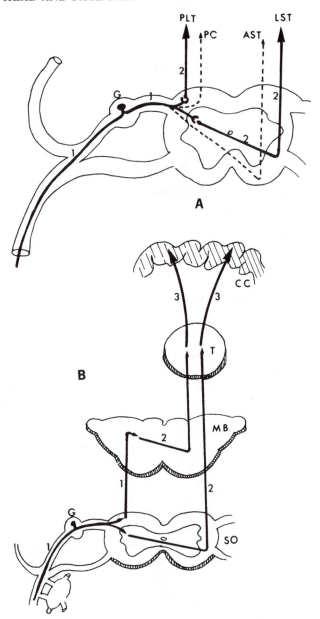

Figure 11–14. Neuron pathways of pain.

(A) The course of sensory fibers in a segmental nerve with its ganglion in the dorsal root (G). Upon entrance into the cord, the fibers ascend on the same side in the posterior lateral tract (PLT) and decussate to cross into the lateral spinothalamic tract; 2 indicates secondary neurons. The posterior column (PC) transmits position sense; AST conveys tactile sensation. (B) 1 = first-stage neurons to the cord; 2 = second-stage neurons through the midbrain (MB) into the thalamus (T); 3 = third-stage neurons, the thalamocortical pathways to the cerebral cortex (CC). (From Cailliet, R: Shoulder Pain, ed 3. FA Davis, Philadelphia, 1991, p 232, with permission.)

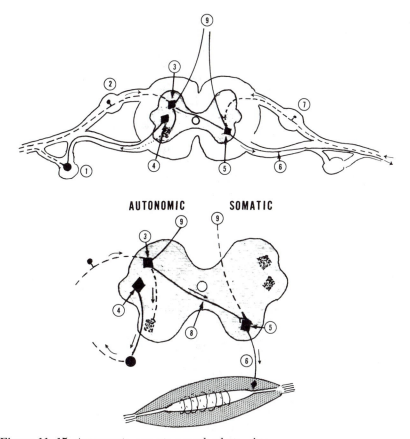

Figure 11–15. Autonomic-somatic neural relationship.

At the cord level the sympathetic fibers *(1)* enter the afferent nerve fibers to accompany the C fibers of the dorsal root ganglion *(2)* then on to the dorsal horn *(3)*. There is a neuronal connection with the intermedial nerve ganglion *(4)* which is the motor sympathetic root *(efferent)*.

There is postulated to be a neural connection *(8)* with the anterior horn cell *(5)* which is motor *(alpha fibers)* to the extrafusal muscle fibers *(6)*. Sensation to the cortex via the thalamic system is through the fibers noted *(9)*.

insofar as pain production is concerned. However, with the sensitized WDR region, these normal mechanoreceptive impulses now elicit pain. Light touch is now painful. These ultimately react with internal neurons that affect the lateral horns of the dorsal root wherein lie the nerve bodies of the afferent sympathetic fibers.

This last neuronal circuit explains the somatic-autonomic relationship (Fig. 11–15) that results in dystrophic and numerous vasomotor reactions of the regions innervated by those specific nerves.

As concurrent muscle spasm frequently accompanies many pain syn-

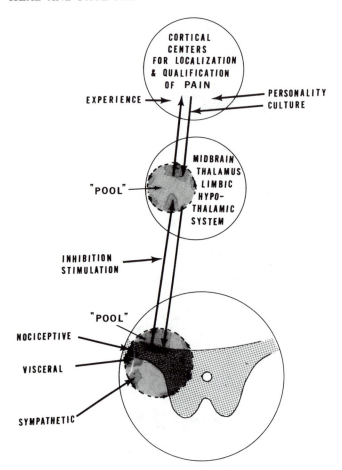

Figure 11–16. Pool of sensory centers in modulation of pain.

From the periphery the first pool is at the gray matter of the dorsal horn of the cord. Ascending there from the midbrain and ultimately the cortical centers. The details are discussed in the text.

dromes and even accentuates the pain with addition of a secondary site of noxious stimulation, the sympathetic-somatic relationship may also be incorporated into this framework.

In summary there are essentially three pools of neuronal modification of pain from the periphery through the dorsal root into the dorsal horn of the cord (Fig. 11–16). The second pool is at the midbrain level, and the third exists at the cortex where pain is localized and qualified.

REFERENCES

1. Woolf, CJ: Evidence for a central component of post-injury pain hypersensitivity. Nature 306:686–688, 1983.
2. Dunner, R: Neuronal plasticity and pain following peripheral tissue inflammation or nerve injury. In Bond, M, Charlton, E, and Woolf, CJ (eds): Proceedings of the Sixth World Congress on Pain, Vol 5, Pain Research and Clinical Management. Elsevier, Amsterdam, 1991, pp 263–276.
3. Wall, PD: The prevention of postoperative pain. Pain 33:289–290, 1988.
4. Dubner, R: Specialization in nociceptive pathways: Sensory discrimination, sensory modulation and neuronal connectivity. In Fields, HL, Dubner, R, and Cervero, F (eds): Advances in Pain Research and Therapy, Vol 9. Raven Press, New York, 1985, pp 111–133.
5. Light, AR and Perl, ER: Reexamination of the dorsal root projection to the spinal dorsal horn including observations on the differential termination of coarse and fine fibers. J Comp Neurol 186:117–132, 1979.
6. Fields, HL and Basbaum, AI: Brainstem control of spinal pain-transmission neurons. Annu Rev Physiol 40:217–248, 1978.
7. Bowsher, D: Pain mechanisms in man. Res Staff Phys 29(12):26–34, 1983.
8. Rexed, B: A cytoarchitectonic atlas of the spinal cord in the cat. J Comp Neurol 100:297, 1954.
9. Selzer, M and Spencer, WA: Convergence of visceral and cutaneous afferent pathways in the lumbar spinal cord. Brain Res 14:331–348, 1969.
10. Aihara, Y, Nakamura, H, Sato, A, and Simpson, A: Neural control of gastric motility with special reference to cutaneo-gastric reflexes. In Brooks, C, et al (eds): Integrative Functions of Autonomic Nervous System. Elsevier, New York, 1979, pp 38–49.
11. Davies, SN and Lodge, D: Evidence for involvement of N-methylaspartate receptors in "wind-up" of class 2 neurons in the dorsal horn of the rat. Brain Res 424:402–406, 1987.
12. Salt, TE and Hill, RG: Pharmacological differentiation between responses of rat medullary dorsal horn neurons to noxious mechanical and noxious thermal cutaneous stimuli. Brain Res 263:167–171, 1983.
13. Woolf, CJ and Thompson, SWN: The induction and maintenance of central sensitization is dependant on N-methyl-aspartic acid receptor activation: Implications for the treatment of post-injury pain hypersensitivity states. Pain 44:293–299, 1991.
14. Mersky, H: Classification of chronic pain: Description of chronic pain syndromes and definitions. Pain (Suppl)3:S1–S225, 1986.
15. Melzak, R: Advances in Neurology, Vol 4. Raven Press, New York, 1974, pp 275–280.
16. Cailliet, R: Shoulder Pain, ed 3. FA Davis, Philadelphia, 1991, pp 227–235.
17. Perroncito, A: La rigenerazione delle fibre nervose. Boll Soc Med Clin Pavia 4:434, 1905.
18. Devor, M: Nerve pathophysiological and mechanisms of pain in causalgia. J Auton Nerv Syst 7:371, 1983.
19. Ecker, A: Norepinephrine in reflex sympathetic dystrophy: An hypothesis. Clin J Pain 5:313, 1989.
20. Perl, ER: Pain and perception. Handbook of Physiology, American Physiological Society, Bethesda, MD, 1984, pp 915–975.
21. Sawehenko, PE and Swanson, LW: The organization of nonadrenergic pathways from the brainstem to the paraventricular and supraoptic nuclei in the rat. Brain Res Rev 4:275–325, 1982.
22. Kalin, NH and Dawson, G: Neuroendocrine dysfunction in depression: Hypothalamic-anterior pituitary systems. Trends in Neurosci 9:261–266, 1986.
23. Ganong, W: The stress response: A dynamic overview. Hosp Pract 23(6):155–190, 1988.
24. Stokes, PE and Sikes, CR: The hypothalamic-pituitary-adrenocortical axis in major depression. Endocr Metabol Clinics NA 17:1–19, 1988.
25. Roberts, WJ: A hypothesis on the physiological basis for causalgia and related pains. Pain 24:297, 1986.

CHAPTER 12

Management of Head and Face Pain

With the concept of pain and its modulation being more precise in neurophysiological and neuropharmacological aspects, the management of pain requires consideration of all of these aspects. In previous chapters, specific treatment modalities and medications for the different types of head and face pain have been discussed.

Pain in the head constitutes a major site of pain complaint.[1] Though sometimes a forecaster of potentially ominous intracranial pathology, the vast majority of headaches present disabling symptoms with no discernible pathology. Basic research has revealed fundamentally neurophysiological and neurohormonal mechanisms that respond to neuropharmacological treatments. Migraine, migraine variant, and cluster headaches make up only a small proportion of headache complaints. The vast majority of headaches are considered tension headaches, implying a muscular substrate.[2] The involved muscles are those of the pericranium. "Tension" appears to be emotional or postural in origin. No precise frequency statistics are available, yet as much as 3 percent of the population may incur a daily tension headache, and 10 percent a weekly headache.

The muscular basis of these tension headaches has been questioned, as electromyographic studies failed to substantiate sustained muscular contraction. The effectiveness of antidepressant medication and other psychotropic drugs in preventing recurrent tension headaches implies a strong if not essential psychogenic basis for the tension.[3]

Pressure research studies indicated that patients suffering tension headaches had a lowered pain tolerance.[4] These studies did not, however, relate to anxiety and hidden depression.[5]

The peripheral mechanisms of headaches, including the muscles, blood vessels, and associated peripheral nervous systems (autonomic and somatic), are no longer considered primary, but are instead giving way to the finding of central nervous involvement. A recently advocated model postulates that, in some cases, the nociceptive afferent impulses are being monitored centrally.[6] Peripheral and central pathways both undoubtedly exist, but their role requires further elucidation.[7]

The proposed vascular-supraspinal-myogenic (VSM) model for pain lays a foundation for further understanding of general pain mechanisms that have a similar basis in other neuromuscular-vascular pain syndromes.[8]

Between 10 and 20 percent of the general population get headaches.[9] Numerous etiologies have been invoked, including blood platelet disorder,[10] cerebrovascular spasm,[11] and central dysnociception.[12] The latter remains a vague concept not satisfactorally explaining the basis of the specific headache.

Recent studies in head and face pain imply central processing of the nociceptive afferent impulses rather than mere ascension of these impulses through the accepted neural pathways transmitting pain. A more precise relationship of tension headaches and myofascial pain with "vascular" headaches is becoming apparent.

Migraine has been divided into two main subtypes: those with and without aura. The classic symptoms of migraine without aura are recurrent "pulsating" unilateral headache lasting 4 to 72 hours, with associated nausea, photophobia, or phonophobia. The migraine with aura is similar. Onset is heralded by a visual aura, gradual spread of neurological (hemiplegic) paresthesia, hypalgesia, and/or paresis. Tension headaches are characterized by episodes of mild to moderate pain described as generalized "pressing," "tightening," or "pressure." The duration varies but may ultimately become constant.

Most if not all of the above types of headache are associated with psychosocial or emotional stress.[13] It has been confirmed that many patients suffering intractable migraine respond favorably to inpatient care, away from irritating events, with mere use of aspirin and antinausea medication (unpublished data by Olesen).

Assuming the totality of the VSM model, all aspects must be addressed and are implied in this model. The vasomotor component of headache postulated by its pulsating characteristics, aggravation by physical activity, and response to vasoactive medications and local vascular compression has been further verified by regional cerebral blood flow (rCBF) studies. These and angiography studies have revealed regions of flow reduction originating posteriorly and spreading anteriorly at a rate of 2 to 6 mm/min.[14] This is followed by hyperfusion hours after the initial phase of diminished flow.[15]

The intracranial and extracranial blood vessels are surrounded by dense meshworks of nerve fibers.[16] Many are sympathetic nerves containing noradrenalin (NA) and neuropeptide Y (NPY). The parasympathetic nerves contain acetylcholine (ACh) and vasoactive polypeptide (VIP). There are other nociceptive peptides, such a substance P and neurokinin (NKA), located within the trigeminal nerve ganglion. The wide dynamic range (WDR) neurons of the trigeminal ganglion have connections to the intracranial and extracranial blood vessels. Noxious stimulation of the pericranial myofascial tissues excite similar neurons.[17] This innervation of myofascial tissue, together with the vascular innervation, may explain the clinical relationship of migraine headaches with myofascial and muscular tension headaches.

This vascular mechanism has become accepted, but the neurophysiological basis for the vasomotor reaction has not been confirmed, nor has its relationship to the muscular component been explained. The proposed VSM model for this reaction is a pathophysiological disturbance initiated by algogenic substances activated by pial arterial nociceptors and affecting the cerebral cortex: a neurovascular mechanism.

The related tenderness of the pericranial muscles that accompanies migraine[18] is also included in this model. Trigger point injections have aborted migraine headaches,[19] as has biofeedback, indicating a direct relationship. Mere muscle tension (sustained contraction) has not been confirmed, as EMG studies are not confirmatory.[20] The concept of the VSM model is that myogenic nociceptor impulses also are involved in the cerebral mechanism.

The cerebral aspect of the VSM model that inhibits the effects of the afferent nociceptor impulses is the basis of this concept. Animal experiments have been performed but as yet have not been confirmed in humans. Decerebration in animals which disconnect cortical aspects have permitted strong facilitory spinal neuron transmission to proceed uninhibited.[21] The on cells of the ventromedial medulla have also been shown to be facilitated.[22] (This material is reviewed in Chapter 1. See also Cailliet.[23])

The VSM model proposed by Olesen does not repudiate the treatment of migraine by vasoactive medication. Rather, it includes the rationale for myofascial intervention and explains the emotional component of headache (see Figs. 12–1 and 12–2). The trigeminal caudalis neuron (TCN) normally transmits input from all the blood vessels indicated as well as the pericranial musculature. Once sensitized it enhances impulses that otherwise would not be sensitive and thus pain-producing. Current concepts indicate that the primary nociception in migraine arises from the vascular system but all sources of input compete within the caudalis neuron modulating via excitatory (EN) or inhibitory (IN) which becomes predominant.

In this model the emotions via the limbic system play a role and the peripheral nociception arises from vasoactive blood vessels as well as the myofascial sites. In migraine, the blood vessels are predominant, and in tension headaches the myofascial input predominates. All may be related in some headaches. Treating head and face pain with this model as a basis indicates that the peripheral mechanisms must be approached, the neurovascular aspects addressed, and all the psychosocial emotional aspects also considered.

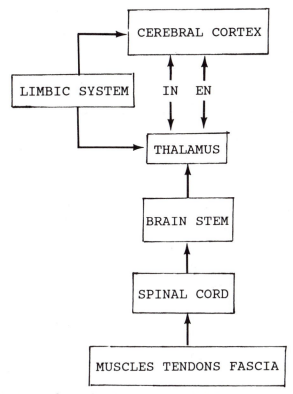

Figure 12–1. Accepted neural pathways of musculoskeletal pain.

The currently accepted pathways of nociceptors from musculoskeletal sites is depicted. The modulation of this pain occurs at the thalamic level with central excitatory *(IN)* and inhibitory *(EN)* input influencing the ultimate degree of experienced pain. The emotional aspects of pain are incurred from limbic system input.

In approaching the peripheral aspects of head and face pain, we need to pay attention to the vascular effects of the presumed trauma. The nociceptor substances allegedly released or created at the local site—vascular, cutaneous tissues or underlying musculature with a neurovascular component—can be easily and effectively diminished by the local application of ice.[24] This nociceptor is possibly histaminelike in its composition and action.

The component muscular aspect of pain is also reduced by the application of ice apparently because of its effect upon the spindle system. "Cooling" has been considered to affect the activity of the low-threshold mechanoreceptors which suppress pain.[25]

Local cryotherapy also has value in suppressing pain of the facial neuralgias as well as in treating myofascial pain (Chapter 7), cervicogenic pain (Chapter 6), posttraumatic pain syndromes (Chapter 8), and temporomandibular joint pain (Chapter 10).

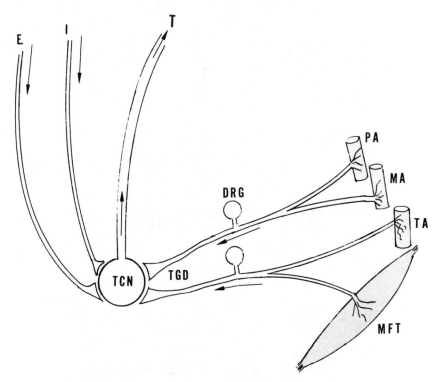

Figure 12–2. Myofascial supraspinal vascular model of pain pathways.

The input into the pain neural pathways are depicted in this MSV model. The afferent impulses originating from the pial arteries *(PA)*, meningeal arteries *(MA)*, and the temporal arteries *(TA)*, compete with the nociceptive impulses of the myofascial tissues *(MFT)*.

All impulses converge through their dorsal root ganglia *(DRG)* to the trigeminal ganglion *(1st)* division nucleus *(TCN)*. Modulation of these impulses that ultimately enter the thalamus *(T)* occurs from descending excitory *(E)* and inhibitory *(I)* fibers from cortical levels.

The local use of heat, preferably moist for its deeper tissue penetration, is of value after, and occasionally in place of, ice. The vasomotor reaction of heat causes a diffusion of the accumulated nociceptor agents and also diminishes the concurrent muscle spasm.

Local treatment of trigger points by injections, ice, and stretch techniques have been discussed in previous chapters and will not be specifically repeated here. They need to be considered and treated whenever they are found to be pertinent in the specific pain syndrome.

BIOFEEDBACK

Sustained muscle contraction ("tension") that initiates or aggravates the pain syndrome can be modified by many techniques. Biofeedback has proven effective.[26] Biofeedback often reproduces the precise pain, providing electromyographic documentation of muscle contraction through surface electrodes on the painful muscles. Biofeedback may also document vasomotor reaction contributing to the underlying pain mechanisms.[27] Simply stated, the concept of biofeedback is to make the patient conscious of muscle tension and bring it under the voluntary control of the patient.

The assumption that sustained muscle contraction is a major cause of pain is generally accepted, although there remains controversy. Recent studies of jaw pain and local tenderness from repeated sustained voluntary muscle contraction failed to produce muscle pain.[28] The advocates of pain occurring from sustained muscle contraction have attributed the sustained muscular contraction to deep-seated emotional tension.

TENS

Transcutaneous electrical nerve stimulation (TENS) has proven effective for intractable pain. TENS has been well accepted in the management of pain and its basis for success has been attributed to the neurophysiological gate concept of pain modulation. Because large-diameter myelinated nerves transmit mechanoreceptor impulses rather than pain nociception, they carry inhibitor impulses that moderate activator impulses and have a lower electrical threshold than unmyelinated fibers that inhibit (modulate) nociceptor activator impulses at the dorsal root and dorsal horn level.

These large mechanoreceptor fibers transmit at a faster speed than do the nociceptor unmyelinated fibers, and when they arrive "ahead" at the "gate" they modulate the pain-producing impulses that enter the dorsal horn through the unmyelinated fibers. This nerve impulse modulation at the dorsal horn diminishes and even obliterates pain.

Although the precise mechanism of TENS remains controversial, TENS has simulated narcotic agents and implied a similar neural (pharmacological) mechanism. High-intensity, low-frequency impulses of less than 10 Hz have resulted in long-lasting analgesia. This benefit has been reversed by naloxone, implying endorphin release by the TENS.[28,29] Electrical stimulation has been shown to increase levels of dopamine and serotonin as well as levels of norepinephrine, which play a role in analgesia.[31]

An inhibition of the spinothalamic tract transmission has also been demonstrated that has not been inhibited by naloxone,[32] therefore making its efficacy neurological as well as pharmacological. Electrical stimulation has been shown to decrease the nerve action potential of α-delta nerves,[33] which

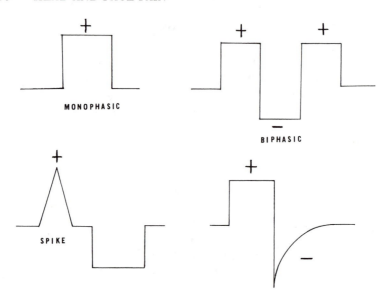

Figure 12–3. Waveforms of TENS.

are accepted as mediators of nociceptor impulse. All these facts need to be assimilated and clarified, as it is well accepted that low-intensity, high-frequency impulses (greater than 50 Hz), which is the standard dosage of the average clinical TENS units, give short-term analgesia and this analgesia is not naloxone-reversible.[34]

Application of TENS in an injured nerve has been most effective if the current is applied proximal to the injury. Its efficacy, however, requires careful monitoring as to the precise site of application, type of current wave length and form (see Figs. 12–3 and 12–4). Many TENS failures have resulted from using a less-than-optimum site of application. Its effective use demands finding the best site, duration, and type of application. TENS is also a modality that enhances other forms of treatment (Fig. 12–5). In patients with chronic pain efficacy of TENS has varied from 12 to 60 percent of patients,[35] but patients with significant depressive illness compounding the pain have a significantly lesser degree of benefit. Hence, TENS cannot be considered a psychotherapeutic modality but is related more to neurogenic and endorphin-related benefit.

A recent article by an oral surgeon advocates and explains the mechanism for success of using ultra-low-frequency TENS.[36] The frequency advocated is 0.66 Hz. This is based on the finding that with frequencies of less than 1 Hz there is significant muscle relaxation.[37] Assuming that muscle tension is a factor if not the major cause of orofacial pain, by releasing muscle tension there is greater clearing of metabolic by-products with the increased blood flow and production of endogenous opioids.[38] Low-frequency TENS

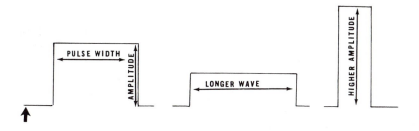

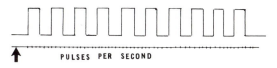

Figure 12–4. Characteristics of TENS application.

does not result in immediate diminution of pain, but after a 20-minute application there is usually a 6- to 8-hour period of relief of pain. Different equipment is required.*

PSYCHOTROPIC MEDICATIONS

Many pain patients are also depressed and their depression intensifies if not initiates their reaction to pain. Therefore the use of psychotropic drugs in the treatment of pain is becoming more prominent.

The effectiveness of tricyclic drugs may be related to their central nervous system effect upon the biogenic amines such as serotonin (5-hydroxy-

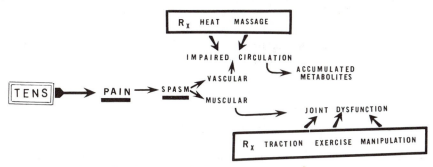

Figure 12–5. Beneficial effects of TENS in treating pain.

---

*The equipment required is BNS-40, registered trademark of Myotronics Inc., 720 Olive Way, Suite 800, Seattle WA 98101.

tryptamine)[39] and norepinephrine. There is evidence that serotonin and norepinephrine-containing neurons are an integral part of the endorphin-mediated pain-modulating system. As many psychotropic drugs block the reuptake of serotonin, this may be the mechanism of pain modulation.

Phenothiazines as an adjunct to narcotic analgesics have a definite benefit when used in conjunction with opiates where they alone are not significantly analgesic. They appear to have value in enhancing the efficacy of tricyclic medication.

Unfortunately, opiates have been inadequately used because of fear of addiction and lack of knowledge and experience in the proper dosage and side effects. Opium receptors have been located in the dorsal horn, which accepts opiates administered locally with no side influences.

CHRONIC PAIN

Patients may experience certain benefits to pain: attention, avoidance of stressful situations, and economic advantages.[40] We pay attention to patients with pain. Patients are conveniently excused from doing things they otherwise could do. They essentially receive more attention than they otherwise would, and subconsciously this may be their desire. Avoidance of stressful situations is possible if there is pain and illness. There is thus also a reduction of anxiety. Finally, economic advantage is society's most costly experience as is apparent in the injured worker who benefits financially and is nonproductive during the illness. Volumes of literature have been written regarding this economic loss to society.[41]

The multidisciplined pain clinic has emerged using behavioral methods,[42] hypnosis,[43] biofeedback, physical therapy, and counseling as well as all medications previously mentioned.

Somatization has been postulated by George Becker,[44] in which the patient expresses in symptoms and with body language what is considered to be an appropriate reaction to pain. There may or may not be a significant underlying physical condition and the symptoms are frequently out of proportion to the underlying condition.

Adults who have been emotionally deprived in their childhood harbor latent emotional needs which becomes evident by somatizing their current complaints. Death in the family, marital turmoil, separation, divorce, etc. all cause somatization which becomes acceptable where a psychological basis is unacceptable. Overuse of medication and alcoholism become evident to the observant examiner. Often the chronic headache patient who fails to improve or benefit becomes the "hateful" patient to the physician.[45] These patients are termed manipulative, demanding, help rejectors, and clingers. They are dreaded by their physician and their care suffers.

REFERENCES

1. Cailliet, R: Head and Face Pain. FA Davis, Philadelphia, 1992 (pending).
2. Ad Hoc Committee on Classification of Headache: Classification of headache. JAMA 179:717–718, 1962.
3. Headache Classification Committee of the International Headache Society: Classification and diagnostic criteria for headache disorders, cranial neuralgias and facial pain. Cephalalgia (Suppl 7) 8:1–96, 1988.
4. Langemark, M, Jensen, K, Jensen, TS, and Olesen, J: Pressure pain thresholds and thermal nociceptive thresholds in chronic tension-type headache. Pain 38:203–210, 1989.
5. Olesen, J and Jensen, R: Getting away from simple muscle contraction as a mechanism of tension-type headache. Pain 46:123–124, 1991.
6. Schoenen, J: Tension-type headache: Pathophysiological evidence for disturbance of "limbic" pathways to the brain stem. Headache 30:314–315, 1990.
7. Olesen, J and Langemark, M: Mechanisms of tension headache. A speculative hypothesis. In Olesen, J and Edvinson, L (eds): Basic Mechanisms of Headache. Elsevier, Amsterdam, 1988, pp 457–461.
8. Olesen, J: Clinical and pathophysiological observations in migraine and tension-type headache explained by integration of vascular, supraspinal and myofascial inputs. Pain 46:125–132, 1991.
9. Rasmussen, BK, Jensen, R, Schroll, M, and Olesen, J: Epidemiology of headache in a serial population—a prevalence study. Pain 46:125–132, 1991.
10. Hannington, E, Jones, RJ, Amess, JA, and Wachowicz, B: Migraine: A platelet disorder. Lancet 720–723, 1981.
11. Wolff, HG: Headache and Other Head Pain. Oxford University Press, New York, 1963.
12. Sicuteri, F: Migraine, a central biochemical dysnociception. Headache 16:145–149, 1986.
13. Henryk-Gutt, R and Rees, WL: Psychological aspects of migraine. J Psychosom Res 17:141–153, 1973.
14. Lauritzen, M, Skyhoj-Olsen, T, Lassen, NA, and Paulson, OB: The changes of regional cerebral blood flow during the course of classical migraine attacks. Ann Neurol 13:633–641, 1983.
15. Wolff, HG: Headache and Other Head Pain. Oxford University Press, New York, 1963.
16. Edvinsson, L, MacKenzie, ET, McCulloch, J, and Uddmann, R: Nerve supply and receptor mechanisms in intra- and extra-cerebral blood vessels. In Olesen, J and Edvinsson, L (eds): Basic Mechanisms of Headache. Elsevier, Amsterdam, 1988, pp 129–144.
17. Sessle, BJ, Hu, JW, Amano, N, and Zhong, G: Convergence of cutaneous, tooth pulp, visceral, neck muscle afferents onto nociceptive and non-nociceptive neurons in trigeminal subnucleus caudalis (medullary dorsal horn) and its implications for referred pain. Pain 27:219–235, 1986.
18. Tfelt-Hansen, P, Lous, I, and Olesen, J: Prevalence and significance of muscle tenderness during common migraine attacks. Headache 21:49–54, 1981.
19. Olesen, J: Some clinical features of the acute migraine attack. An analysis of 750 patients. Headache 18:268–271, 1978.
20. Bakke, M, Tfelt-Hansen, P, Olesen, J, and Moller, E: Action of some pericranial muscles during provoked attacks of common migraine. Pain 14:121–135, 1982.
21. Hillman, P and Wall, PD: Inhibitory and excitatory factors controlling lamina 5 cells. Exp Brain Res 9:284–306, 1969.
22. Fields, HL and Heinricher, M: Brainstem modulation of nociceptor-driven withdrawal reflexes. Ann NY Acad Sci 563:34–44, 1989.
23. Cailliet, R: Chronic pain: Is it necessary? Arch Phys Med 60:1979.
24. Lehmann, JF and DeLateur, BJ: Therapeutic cold. Diathermy and superficial heat, laser

and cold therapy. In Krusen's Handbook of Physical Medicine and Rehabilitation, ed 4, Kottke, FJ and Lehmann, JF (eds): WB Saunders, Philadelphia, 1990, pp 340–350.

25. Bini, G, Cruccu, G, Hagbarth, KE, Schady, W, and Torebjork, E: Analgesic effect of vibration and cooling on pain induced by intraneural electrical stimulation. Pain 18:239–248, 1984.

26. Birk, L: Behavioral Medicine: Seminars in Psychiatry. Grune & Stratton, New York, 1973.

27. Gaarder, KR, et al: Clinical Biofeedback: A Procedural Manual. Williams & Wilkins, Baltimore, 1977.

28. Clark, GT, Adler, RC, and Lee JJ: Jaw pain and tenderness levels during and after repeated sustained maximal voluntary protrusion. Pain 45:17–22, 1991.

29. Sjolund, BH, and Eriksson, MBE: The influence of naloxone on analgesia produced by peripheral conditioning stimulation. Brain Res 173:295–301, 1979.

30. Salar, G, Job, I, Mingrino, S, et al: Effect of transcutaneous electrotherapy on CSF B-endorphine content in patients without pain problems. Pain 10:169–172, 1981.

31. Akil, H and Liebskind, JC: Monoaminergic mechanisms of stimulation produced analgesia. Brain Res 94:279–296, 1975.

32. Chung, JM, et al: Prolonged inhibition of primate spinothalamic tract cells by peripheral nerve stimulation. Pain 19:259–275, 1984.

33. Ignelzi, RJ and Nyquist, JK: Direct effect of electrical stimulation on peripheral nerve evoked activity: Implications in pain relief. J Neurosurg 45:159–165, 1976.

34. Loeser, J, Black, R, and Christman, A: Relief of pain by transcutaneous stimulation. J Neurosurg 42:308–314, 1975.

35. Long, DM and Hagfors, N: Electrical stimulation in the nervous system: The current status of electrical stimulation of the nervous system for the relief of pain. Pain 1:109–123, 1975.

36. Langberg, GJ: Ultra-low-frequency TENS: A well-kept secret. Pain Management Sept–Oct:278–280, 1990.

37. Dixon, HH and Dickel, HA: Tension headache. Northwest Med 66:817–820, 1967.

38. Sjolund, BH and Eriksson, MBE: Endorphins and Analgesia Produced by Peripheral Conditioning Stimulation. Vol 3, Advances in Pain Research and Therapy. Raven Press, New York, 1979.

39. Besson, JM: Serotonin and Pain. In Besson, JM (ed): International Congress Series 879. Elsevier, Amsterdam, 1990.

40. Unikel, IP: How we learn chronic pain and sickness. In Brena, SF (ed): Chronic Pain: America's Hidden Epidemic. Atheneum/SMI, New York, 1978, pp 19–26.

41. Pain and Disability: Clinical, Behavioral and Public Policy Perspectives, Institute of Medicine: Osterweis, M, Kleinman, A, and Mechanics, D (eds), National Academy Press, Washington DC, 1987.

42. Fordyce, WE: Behavioral Methods for Chronic Pain and Illness. CV Mosby, St Louis, 1976.

43. Hilgard, ER and Hilgard, JR: Hypnosis in the Relief of Pain. Kaufmann, Los Altos, CA, 1975.

44. Becker, GE: Personal communication.

45. Groves, JE: Taking care of the hateful patient. N Engl J Med 298(16):883–887, 1978.

CHAPTER 13

Psychological Testing in Patients with Chronic Pain

Objective documentation, verification, and quantification of the emotional and psychological aspects influencing complaints of pain, especially chronic complaints, in a patient with minimal objective findings, remains a significant concern to practitioners treating the patient with pain. Numerous tests are reported in the literature almost daily.

There are several potential uses for psychological testing:[1]

1. Routine screening of patients whose pain complaints seem to have a large psychological component
2. Confirmation of a psychiatric diagnosis
3. Acquisition of a basis for appropriate treatment protocol
4. Initiation of a research program

Only some of these tests will be discussed. It must be stated that any test must be carefully used to diagnose a patient with pain. The initial assumption of a psychological basis for the pain must have validity and the treatment, as well as the diagnosis, cannot be based solely on the outcome of the test. Treatment that ensues from the interpretation of any test must also rely upon the age, sex, cultural background, educational level, potential secondary gains including economic (from litigation), and the competence of the therapist.

A test that has had acceptance for years is the Minnesota Multiphasic Personality Inventory (MMPI) (Fig. 13–1).[2] This test is a self-administered true-false test and consists of a 550-question form or an abbreviated 399-question form. The test is computer-scored and interpreted. It is a checklist

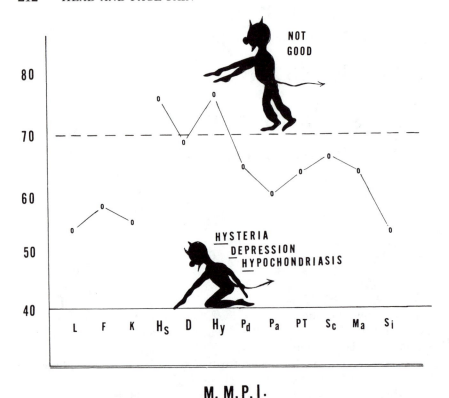

M. M. P. I.

Figure 13–1. Minnesota Multiphasic Personality Inventory (MMPI).

of physical and emotional symptoms and involves the symptoms of the present (the time of the examination) as well as the past.

Scores vary in patients with acute versus chronic pain. In the (chronic) latter, patients score higher in hypochondriasis (HS), depression (D), and hysteria (Hy), whereas patients with acute pain score higher in hypochondriasis (HS) and hysteria (Hy). As both acute and chronic pain patients are preoccupied with the significance of their pain they express agitation (elevated Ma score), which drops when the pain becomes chronic and depression (D) rises.

The original population sample for the MMPI was 700 men and women, all white and residents of Minnesota. The average members of the group interviewed were semiskilled workers or farmers with an eighth-grade education. The phrasing of the statements was also considered awkward and not clear. Many topics such as drug abuse, alcoholism, and suicidal tendencies were not addressed. The revised MMPI-2 corrected these flaws and now consists of 567 items; it includes a posttraumatic stress scale and a gender role scale and is being re-evaluated as to its efficacy.[3]

In evaluating an MMPI scale one cannot determine whether the scales were elevated prior to or as a result of the chronic pain.[4] Another disadvantage to the MMPI is the time needed for the patient to perform the test and the different interpretations placed on it by psychologists.

The Eysenck personality test (EPI) measures stability versus neuroticism and introversion versus extroversion.[5] This test basically indicates the stability of the patient's reaction to stress and the tendency for the patient to break down. There is a direct relationship of susceptibility to the N score. A high N does not indicate neuroticism but merely susceptibility and indicates an introverted person. Extroverts allegedly complain more freely than do introverts but have a higher threshold to pain. The EPI test is not as much help in therapy as it is in evaluating the patient's susceptibility to decompensate under stress.

The Beck Depression Inventory[6] consists of 21 items; it is self-administered and can be executed in 5 minutes. Each item relates to a factor regarding depression but not other psychological factors aggravating pain.

Hendler has propounded an excellent test validating the complaint of chronic pain, but it has been utilized essentially for low back pain.[7] Its validity for head and face pain, pending successful outcome from surgical intervention as noted in low back pain, remains untested.

It is apparent that there is a strong emotional component of any face and head pain and the proportion frequently remains obscure, often to the detriment of the patients and the frustration of the therapist. Cultural and educational factors in today's society imply potential ominous sequelae of any pain in that region.

The International Association for the Study of Pain and the American Psychiatric Association both have classified orofacial pain of psychogenic origin with the former claiming that orofacial pain is psychogenic only if no known physical cause or pathofunction can account for the pain and if contributing factors are undeniably present.[8] The American Psychiatric Association originally classified orofacial pain as a "psychogenic pain disorder" and later defined it as a "somatoform pain disorder."[9,10]

With these claims and implications it is evident that many facial and head pains, being subjective complaints, with little if any confirmatory objective findings, tend to be labeled psychogenic. Failure of the patient to respond to what is considered "appropriate" treatment lends further support to a psychogenic rather an organic etiology. Accusation rather than diagnosis results and pain becomes chronic and intractable. The frustrated patient may then pursue inappropriate exotic treatments.

Patient-physician rapport and communication are the crux of appropriate examination, diagnosis, and treatment. Listening to the complaint and interpreting it properly is the initial basis of diagnosis and the beginning of effective treatment. The examiner should have knowledge of the presence of an underlying psychological aspect of any, if not all, pain complaints, especially in evaluating orofacial-head pain.

The use of understandable words in explaining the cause and effects of a patient's pain is mandatory. It can never be denied that a patient's cooperation in receiving benefit from any treatment begins with a clear understanding of the problem. The presence of a psychological component to the acceptance of pain—either as causative or as an aggravation—can and must be portrayed to the patient. Its acceptance is the beginning of relief and even cure.

REFERENCES

1. Rome, HP, Harness, DM, and Kaplan, HJ: Psychological and behavioral aspects of chronic facial pain. In Jacobson, AL and Donlon, WC (eds): Headache and Facial Pain. Raven Press, New York, 1990.
2. Dahlstrom, WG, Welsh, GS, and Dahlstrom, LE: An MMPI Handbook, Vol 1. University of Minnesota Press, Minneapolis, 1960.
3. Kingsbury, SJ: Why has the MMPI been revised? Harvard Mental Health Letter 7(12):8, 1991.
4. Naliboff, BD, Cohen, MJ, and Yellen, AN: Does the MMPI differentiate chronic illness from chronic pain? Pain 13:333–341, 1982.
5. Bond, MR: Pain: Its Nature, Analysis and Treatment. Churchill Livingstone, Edinburgh, 1984, pp 45–50.
6. Beck, AT, Ward, CH, Mendelson, M, Mock, J, and Erbaugh, J: Arch Gen Psychiatry 4:561–571, 1961.
7. Hendler, NH: The four stages of pain. In Hendler, NH, Long, DM, and Wise, TN (eds): Diagnosis and Treatment of Chronic Pain. John Wright-PSG Publishing, Boston, 1982.
8. Mersky, H: Classification of chronic pain, descriptions of chronic pain syndromes and definitions of pain terms. Pain (Suppl)3: 1986.
9. American Psychiatric Association: Committee on Nomenclature and Statistical Manual of Mental Disorders, ed 3. American Psychiatric Association, Washington, DC, 1980.
10. American Psychiatric Association Diagnostic and Statistical Manual of Mental Disorders, ed 3 rev. American Psychiatric Association, Washington, DC, 1987.

CHAPTER 14

Clinical Aspects of Depression in Patients with Chronic Pain

Admittedly many patients with chronic pain are depressed, and there are many forms of depression, not all of which are related. The causal relationship remains obscure, and whether depression causes or is the sequela of chronic pain remains unconfirmed.[1]

If chronic pain has resulted in depression the obvious therapeutic approach would be to eliminate or moderate the pain, allowing the depression would ultimately diminish or subside. Depression, however, has also been ascertained as pertinent in causing pain or at least aggravating the disabling symptomatology. In this condition the alleviation of pain may need to be preceded by the moderation or elimination of the depression.

A better understanding of depression is mandated. Unfortunately it may be overlooked or magnified in importance by the examining physician. The manner in which the diagnosis is ascertained and, more important, how it is explained to the patient has often been mismanaged. Pain can cause fatigue, interfere with sleep, and be responsible for disability or even unemployment. It behooves the examining and treating physician to fully understand and recognize the symptoms that lead to the diagnosis of depression and its specific type.

The symptoms of depression are numerous and vary with the individuals. The American Psychiatric Association has documented the criteria of depression (see Table 14–1).

The average physician may not have sufficient knowledge or time to specifically ascertain the degree and type of depression. The need for recognition or its possibility, nevertheless, is obvious so that the condition be addressed and treated.

As noted in Table 14–1, at least five of the symptoms must have been

Table 14–1. DIAGNOSTIC CRITERIA FOR MAJOR DEPRESSIVE EPISODES

A. At least five of the following symptoms have been present during the same 2-week period and represent a change from previous functioning, or at least one of the symptoms is either (1) a depressed mood, or (2) loss of interest or pleasure. (Do not include symptoms that are clearly due to a physical condition, mood-incongruent delusions or hallucinations, incoherence, or marked loosening of association.)

  (1) Depressed mood (or can be irritable mood in children and adolescents) most of the day, nearly every day, as indicated either by subjective account or observation by others

  (2) Markedly diminished interest or pleasure in all, or almost all, activities most of the day, nearly every day, as indicated either by subjective account or observation by others of apathy most of the time

  (3) Significant weight loss or weight gain when not dieting (e.g., more than 5 percent of body weight in a month) or decrease or increase in appetite nearly every day in children (consider failure to make expected weight gains)

  (4) Insomnia or hypersomnia nearly every day

  (5) Psychomotor agitation or retardation nearly every day (observable by others, not merely subjective feelings of restlessness or being slowed down)

  (6) Fatigue or loss of energy every day

  (7) Feelings of worthlessness or excessive or inappropriate guilt (which may be delusional) nearly every day (not merely self-reproach or guilt about being sick)

  (8) Diminished ability to think or concentrate, or indecisiveness, nearly every day (either subjective account or as observed by others)

  (9) Recurrent thoughts of death (not just fear of dying), recurrent suicidal ideation without a specific plan for committing suicide

B. (1) It cannot be established that an organic factor initiated and maintained the disturbance.

  (2) The disturbance is not a normal reaction to the death of a loved one (uncomplicated bereavement). (Morbid preoccupation with worthlessness, suicidal ideation, marked functional impairment or psychomotor retardation of prolonged duration suggest bereavement complicated by major depression.)

C. At no time during the disturbance have there been delusions or hallucinations for as long as 2 weeks in the absence of prominent mood symptoms (i.e., before the mood symptoms developed or after they have remitted).

D. Not superimposed on schizophrenia, schizophreniform disorder, delusional disorder, or psychotic disorder NOS

Source: American Psychiatric Association. Diagnostic and Statistical Manual of Mental Disorders, ed 3 rev. Washington, DC, 1987.

Table 14–2. DIAGNOSTIC CRITERIA FOR BIPOLAR
MANIC EPISODE

A. A distinct period of abnormally and persistently elevated expansive or irritable mood.

B. During the period of mood disturbance, at least three of the following symptoms have persisted (four if the mood is only irritable) and have been present to a significant degree.
(1) Inflated self-esteem or grandiosity
(2) Decreased need for sleep, e.g., feels rested after only 3 hours of sleep
(3) More talkative than usual or pressure to keep talking
(4) Flight of ideas or subjective experience that thoughts are racing
(5) Distractibility, i.e., attention too easily drawn to unimportant or irrelevant external stimuli
(6) Increase in goal-directed activity (either socially, at work or school, or sexually) or psychomotor agitation
(7) Excessive involvement in pleasurable activities which have a high potential for painful consequences, e.g., the person engages in unrestrained buying sprees, sexual indiscretions, or foolish business investments

C. Mood disturbance sufficiently severe to cause marked impairment in occupational functioning or in usual social activities or relationships with others, or to necessitate hospitalization to prevent harm to self or others.

D. At no time during the disturbance have there been delusions or hallucinations for as long as 2 weeks in the absence of prominent mood symptoms (i.e., before the mood symptoms developed or after they have remitted).

E. Not superimposed on schizophrenia, schizophreniform disorder, delusional disorder, or psychotic disorder NOS.

F. It cannot be established that an organic factor initiated and maintained the disturbance (somatic antidepressant treatment, e.g., drugs, ECT) that apparently precipitates a mood disturbance should not be considered an etiological organic factor.

Source: American Psychiatric Association. Diagnostic and Statistical Manual of Mental Disorders, 3 ed rev. Washington, DC, 1987.

present during the same 2-week period and represent a change from previous functioning. These criteria are needed to be diagnostic. The patient must have exhibited a depressed mood and diminished interest or pleasure in all or almost all activities of daily living for those 2 weeks. Often a patient expresses depression but the examining physician fails to notice the hidden depression, with subtle signs and symptoms.

When the patient with chronic pain meets these criteria the diagnosis is apparent, but when the criteria are not met precisely the diagnosis remains obscure. This is the type of patient that taxes the expertise and efficiency of the therapist.

The depressed patient suffering from chronic pain often becomes defensive when questioned about being depressed for fear of being considered crazy. Many patients have been inappropriately approached by their physicians or have been exposed to inaccurate information from newspapers, magazine articles, television programs, or personal contacts.

A structured-interview technique for diagnosing DSM-III-R disorders that is considered reliable has recently been published,[2] but unfortunately it is time-consuming and therefore is usually used only by psychiatrists or psychologists. It appears best, therefore, to make an appropriate referral for further diagnosis in a manner that allies rather than accuses or threatens the patient. The relationship of depression as a contributing or causative factor must also be carefully evaluated.

The distinction between unipolar and bipolar disorders must also be made. The diagnostic criteria for bipolar disorders are outlined in Table 14-2. There are also other categories of diagnostic criteria including melancholic type of depressive episodes, dysthymia, atypical depression, and masked depression. It must also always be remembered that depression may be a sequela of a medical disorder such as central nervous disease, endocrine disorder, etc., or the residual of drug use and withdrawal.

REFERENCES

1. Dworkin, RH and Gitlin, MJ: Clinical aspects of depression in chronic pain patients. Clin J Pain 7:79–94, 1991.
2. Spitzer, RL, Williams, JBW, Gibbon, M, and First, MB: Users guide to the structured clinical interview for DSM-III-R. American Psychiatric Association, Washington, DC, 1990.

Index

An "f" following a page number indicates a figure. A "t" following a page number indicates a table.